Spilling My Guts

A Crohn's Chronicle

RUSS DIMINO

Secret Identity Press

Cover design by Richell Balansag

Interior layout by Abdul Rehman

Author photo by Cora Dimino

ISBN paperback: 979-8-9881200-0-1
ISBN e-book: 979-8-9881200-1-8

https://www.russdimino.com

Names: Dimino, Russ, author.
Title: Spilling my guts : a Crohn's chronicle / Russ Dimino.
Description: [Rochester, New York] : Secret Identity Press, [2023]
Identifiers: ISBN: 979-8-9881200-0-1 (paperback) | 979-8-9881200-1-8 (ebook)
Subjects: LCSH: Dimino, Russ. | Crohn's disease--Patients--United States--Biography. | Crohn's disease--Treatment. | Crohn's disease--Alternative treatment. | LCGFT: Autobiographies.
Classification: LCC: RC862.E52 | DDC: 616.3/440092--dc23

For Dominic and Cora,

Never be afraid to tell a story

that only you can tell

Chapter One

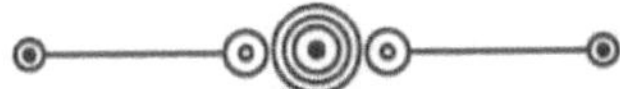

I can still remember the dream I had the night the symptoms first started. In it, I was eating a bowl of cereal. But when I looked down, the cereal was actually a bowl of long, sharp sticks. Repulsed by them, I ran to get something to drink, taking huge gulps of water to wash the cereal-sticks down, only to realize I had just accidentally consumed water from a dirty fish tank. Gripped with nausea, I was certain I was going to throw up.

I woke up from the dream still feeling nauseous, like I really had just eaten sticks and drank dirty fish tank water. Groggy, I got out of bed, the disturbing dream still playing over and over in my mind, intertwined with the sour feeling in my stomach. I made my way to the bathroom. Maybe if I did actually throw up, it would get rid of this awful feeling. Except I didn't need to throw up.

I sat down on the toilet. What came out of me was painful. Violent. Urgent. As if my body was trying to expel poison. There was a sharp pain in my gut, like I really did have sticks in there.

It wasn't diarrhea. Not really. That's an important distinction to make. Most people would hear someone describe an urgent, violent, nauseous experience in the bathroom as diarrhea, but it was different from that. It didn't have the loose, liquidy quality that true diarrhea would have. It was fully formed, but it needed to come out right now. And it hurt.

Something was definitely not right.

It was the summer of 2005, and I was twenty-three years old. I had graduated from the State University of New York at Fredonia with a Bachelor of Arts in Media Arts with a minor in Communications. I'd had grand plans. I was going to be a famous Hollywood filmmaker or screenwriter, maybe work in television. These illustrious career plans had somehow not materialized. I was living with my parents and working part time at Sam's Club in Rochester, New York, as a COS, or check-out supervisor.

As a COS, sometimes my duties involved me going in at six a.m. to help get the club ready to open for business. One morning, not long after the incident I just described, I was driving in for one of those early a.m. opening shifts. With no traffic on the roads at that hour, the drive usually took about twenty minutes. Well, five minutes into the drive, I had a sudden, sharp, twisting feeling in the pit of my stomach. I had to go to the bathroom, and I had to go right now.

I didn't know what to do. If I turned around and went back home, I would definitely end up being late to work. If I kept going, I was 90% sure I was going to shit my pants before I got there. All I could do was keep driving; it didn't make sense to turn around. I was coming up to a gas station. Was it open? I wasn't sure. I envisioned getting out of the car, going into the gas station, and maybe there was no public restroom, or maybe there was one but I'd have to ask an attendant for a key.

I couldn't do it. I didn't stop. All I could do was clench up every muscle in my body, try to stay focused, and try to keep driving. I was running through every scenario possible in my head. It was so early in the morning. Could I pull over to the side of the road and just go on someone's front lawn like an animal? I was starting to think that might be the most rational thing to do— that's how desperate I was becoming. With no one else on the road, I gunned it, speeding toward work as fast as I could.

Somehow, what seemed like an eternity later, bathed in a cold sweat, I pulled into the Sam's Club parking lot. Employees were required to park in an area of the lot farthest away from the building, leaving the prime parking spots for customers. I got out of the car, every fiber of my being trying to keep everything in. I did an awkward straight-legged sprint for the front door, saying a prayer over and over in my head that I was not about to defecate in my pants on my way in to work.

Here's the kicker: At that hour of the day, the doors to Sam's Club were locked because the club was not open yet. Those of us who had to be in prior to the actual hours of operation had to ring a buzzer and wait for a member of management to come open the emergency exit to let us in. Sometimes someone came right way. Sometimes it would take several minutes. As I did my agonizing march to the door, I saw there was a group of at least six or seven employees already gathered outside the door, waiting for someone to open it and let everyone in.

On the one hand, I took it as a good sign. If that many people were waiting to be let in, odds were the buzzer had already been pressed a couple of times. On the other hand, that was no guarantee that the door would be opened anytime soon. Sometimes the only manager with the key to the door was on a forklift or something, getting a pallet down from the steel risers to stock the floor.

As I came up to join the group, I also knew I was going to be incapable of carrying on anything close to a conversation with anyone. Even mild chitchat, a quick "Hi, how are you?" was going to take more mental effort than I was able to spare from my complete and utter focus on keeping from soiling myself.

I leaned against the metal railing that ran alongside the exit and separated the walkway outside the door from the parking lot. I tried to focus on breathing. I tried to focus on staying calm. I tried to focus on not defecating in my pants. This lasted for approximately 1,000 years. It was early enough in the morning that no one really talked to me or paid any attention to me. Everyone was tired, half asleep, grumbling about how long it was taking anyone to come open the door. (Yeah, tell me about it!)

Finally, the universe saw fit to answer my anguished prayers, and the door opened. Everyone filed inside. I levitated off the ground and flew into the building. I had tunnel vision as I homed in on the bathroom like a heat-seeking missile locked in on its target. While everyone else was punching in at the time clock, I was dropping my pants and sitting my shaking ass down on the toilet seat. I didn't even care that I was going to be clocking in late.

I was thankful to God, Jesus, and the Holy Ghost that I hadn't had an accident in my pants upon entering my place of employment.

What resulted was the same nausea-ridden, forceful, painful expulsion from my body as the night of the cereal-stick and fish-water dream.

What was happening to me? Was this a stomach bug that I just couldn't shake? It didn't feel like it, but I had no other concept of what it could even be. Little did I know this was only the beginning of a disease I would fight for years. One that would land me in the hospital multiple times, put me through a ridiculous number of treatments and medications, and ultimately lead to major surgery to remove a considerable amount of my guts.

Chapter Two

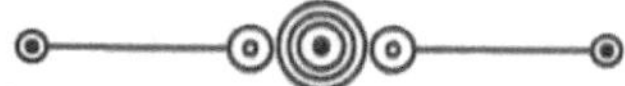

Let's back up a bit so I can introduce someone who is integral to this story. It was October of 2003, and I was attending SUNY Fredonia. There was a big Halloween party at the apartment of my good friends Mike and Jeff, who I had been buddies with since high school. Rap music was playing at full blast on the stereo. A guy dressed as a baby, complete with pacifier and diaper, flirted with a girl dressed as a fairy princess. Morpheus from *The Matrix* was doing shots with Avril Lavigne at the kitchen table, and Lara Croft was funneling a beer in the backyard, being cheered on by Uncle Jesse from *Full House*. I was there dressed as Superman, ready to save the day if the ghosts and goblins got too out of control.

A bunch of us were playing a card game at a table in the middle of the living room when I spotted her. A shy girl dressed as a "lady of the evening" was watching us play cards with quiet interest. She was standing just close enough to laugh at our jokes but not close enough to get pulled into the conversation. Her cautious attention was charming. To be honest, this loud and rambunctious party was not really my scene. I was not a big drinker, and I was much more introverted than most of my buddies. So this cute girl watching us from a careful distance was endearing to me. We caught each other's eye.

"Do you want to play?" I asked.

"Oh, no thanks. I don't know how," she said.

"Do you want to learn?"

"Okay!" She smiled and came over and sat next to me.

It was a simple and sweet connection in the middle of all the wild and crazy revelry.

Her name was Amanda, and she was my friend Pam's roommate. We had been at some of the same group gatherings before, but somehow we had never interacted or paid much attention to each other. Tonight was different though. She had a quiet demeanor, a disarming smile, and bright blue-green eyes. Her gentle shyness in the midst of this raucous party seemed to stop time. It was like we were pulled into our own little bubble, and everything outside of it just became a blur of background noise. I explained the game as we played, not even caring who else heard me narrating what I was about to do. I was playing for an audience of one, and her attention was the prize I wanted to win.

After that night, Amanda and I started hanging out more, usually as part of a larger group of mutual friends. One night in December we were out at a dimly lit, smoke-filled dive bar playing a game of darts. After I took my turn, I walked back over to where Amanda was standing casually beside the wooden railing that separated the small gaming area from the rest of the bar. As I leaned back against the railing, I accidentally placed my hand on top of hers. I didn't pull it away. Neither did she. We ended up holding hands for most of the rest of the night.

We began officially dating in February of 2004. When we told our friends the big news, it was met with confusion. Amanda and I had been so inseparable since the Halloween party that everyone else already assumed we were dating. It was like we were the last ones to know how much we really liked each other.

When we both graduated, we weren't going too far away from each other. Amanda started a music therapy internship at a place in Newark, New York, working with adults with intellectual and developmental disabilities. I moved back home to Rochester with my parents. It was a pretty full house, with me; my dad, Frank; my mom, Linda; my younger sister, Val; my younger brother, Josh; and my grandma Patricia all under one roof.

I picked things back up at my aforementioned COS job at Sam's Club. I had worked there on and off for a few years, mostly over the summers or on breaks from school. It had always been reassuring to know I could come home and get right back on the schedule to pick up some hours and have some money in my bank account each semester. Now that I had graduated, though, I felt stuck. It was nice to have a safety net of gainful employment while I looked for a "real" job. But what did that job look like, and how long would it take to find it?

The drive from my house in Rochester to Amanda's internship in Newark took less than an hour. One of us would make the drive out to see the other about once a week. My hours at Sam's varied a lot; I was not on any kind of set schedule, and my days off were never consistent. Whenever it made sense to do so, I would drive out and stay a night in Newark with her, or she would drive out and crash at my parents' place. She fit right in with my family, with her calm demeanor and cheerful sense of humor. We liked going out to dinner, watching nineties sitcoms like *Full House* and *Boy Meets World*, and listening to the music of Billy Joel, Elton John, Matchbox Twenty, and Barenaked Ladies. Mostly we just loved spending time together.

In the summer of 2005, I was at a comic book convention in Chicago with Mike, flipping through a box of *Incredible Hulk* back issues, trying to fill some gaps in my collection. My cell phone rang. It was Amanda.

"Hey!" I said. "How's it going?"

"Pretty good! You guys having fun at the convention?"

"Yeah, we're having a great time," I said. "I met Margot Kidder earlier today. She signed an autograph for me and everything. It was awesome!"

"Oh wow, that's amazing."

I could tell there was something on her mind. She wasn't calling just to check in.

"Is everything all right?" I asked.

"Oh, yeah, yeah, everything is fine. I just wanted to ask you something. Is this a good time?"

"Sure. What's up, honey?"

"I wanted to ask you… if I took a job in Virginia, would you come with me?"

If this were a movie, there would be a record scratch sound effect here.

"What?"

"There's a music therapy job I want to apply for in Virginia. I think it would be a great opportunity for me. If I moved there, I was wondering if you would come with me."

It was bizarrely surreal. Here I was, at a convention center, hunched over a long box of bagged and boarded back issues, surrounded by fellow nerds and geeks hunting for toys, comics, and autographs. And, much like our first conversation surrounded by fellow college-age revelers at a Halloween party, Amanda and I were having an extremely important personal moment in the midst of a world of chaotic commotion, everyone around us unaware that something momentous was happening.

"Listen," I said, "I need a minute to process that. I'm definitely not saying no. Let's talk more about this when I get home."

After we hung up, Mike came over and asked what was up.

"That was Amanda," I said. "She just asked me to move to Virginia with her."

"Jesus!" Mike exclaimed. "That's a phone call you take at a comic convention?"

I felt bad being so noncommittal in that moment, but it was not a question that I was prepared for. It was a lot to think about. Other than college, I had never lived away from home before. Me and Amanda, on our own in Virginia, not knowing anyone, was an intimidating thought. I wasn't sure I wanted to move away from my family and friends.

On the other hand, I couldn't let Amanda move there all by herself. This was a girl who really understood me, who cared about me, who got me. It's a cliché, but we were totally ourselves around each other. As much as the thought of leaving the only real home I had ever known scared me, I could not stand the idea of being apart from Amanda.

Besides, I didn't exactly have any great career prospects cropping up at home. I was starting to feel embarrassed that I still worked at Sam's Club. Some of my coworkers who knew I had graduated college would ask me how the job search was going, and I always dreaded having to swallow my pride and say that I hadn't found anything yet. I had sent my resume to all of the local TV stations, video production companies, marketing agencies, but no one was biting. I had made follow-up calls to all of them but had yet to land an interview. Maybe getting out of my little corner of the world would present some new opportunities.

Amanda ended up taking the job at a geriatric hospital in Burkeville, Virginia, and I decided to join her. I put in for a transfer to a Walmart in the area, since Sam's Club is owned by the Walmart Corporation. My transfer was accepted. I would be working at the customer service desk at the Blackstone Walmart. It was not exactly a lateral career move. In fact, I would be taking a pay cut. But it was full time, whereas my COS job at Sam's Club was only part time, and I never knew for sure how many hours I would have from week to week. So despite the Walmart job being less pay, it would be a guaranteed forty hours a week, and it would come with health insurance. It was also great just knowing I would have a job waiting for me when I got to Virginia.

The day before I was set to leave for Virginia, I was in my room packing. Amanda was already there, settling into her new job. She was living in a house on the hospital grounds, since part of her employment there came with three months of free housing—a pretty amazing perk.

My dad poked his head in my room and knocked on the open door.

"Need any help?" he asked.

"Nah," I said, cramming a few more things into a box. "I think I've got most of it."

The sight of my partially emptied room seemed to get to him a little bit. He didn't say anything for a long moment as he looked around. There were still posters hanging up, but I'd taken my wall calendar down to bring with me. My bookshelf had vacant spots where I'd grabbed some favorite novels. I'd taken several framed photos off my dresser, but knickknacks from my childhood still remained. My dozen or so boxes full of comic books were staying put, but most of my DVDs were coming with me. It was a room divided.

Dad asked what time I was planning to leave the next day. It was about a nine-hour drive to Burkeville, so I said I was just planning to get up, eat breakfast, and then hit the road. He asked about the place we were staying. From what I had heard from Amanda, it was really nice, a big two-story house. We'd stay rent-free while we looked for more permanent housing.

Out of nowhere, my dad asked, "Do you think you'll marry her?"

The question caught me off guard. I wasn't sure exactly why he was asking. I thought maybe there was an underlying moral question about the fact that I was moving in with a girl that I wasn't married to. Amanda and I had lived together for a semester in college, but that was different, mostly for practical and economic reasons. This was a conscious and deliberate decision to move in together. Still, I wasn't sure if that's what my dad was getting at. Was he just wondering how serious I was about this girl and wanting to make sure that my heart was in the right place? A fair question, since I was about to move to another state to be with her.

I didn't have to think about it very long. Though I was surprised by the question, I was even more surprised by how quickly and easily I was able to answer it. "Yeah," I said. "Yeah, Dad, I think so."

Dad smiled. I'm like my dad in a lot of ways. We are both men of few words. He didn't need to say anything else. He gave me a hug.

The next morning, I loaded up as many worldly possessions as I could fit into my Ford Tempo, waved goodbye to my family, and struck out for Virginia.

It was a long drive, and in the days before smartphones and GPS, I navigated with turn-by-turn directions I had printed out from MapQuest. I made a few stops on the way down, once to get something to eat and several times to avail myself of rest-stop bathrooms. I was still struggling with the urgent need to relieve my bowels at times, so being on the road for a long stretch of time was not ideal. The nine-hour drive ended up taking closer to twelve hours, and it was well after dark by the time I arrived. Amanda ran outside and straight into my arms.

"What took you so long?" she asked with a laugh. "Did you get lost?"

"Hey," I said, holding her tight. "I'm here now. That's the important thing."

The house we were staying in was gorgeous. There were three bedrooms, two full bathrooms, a nice big living room with a fireplace, a dining room, kitchen, everything fully furnished. We were definitely spoiled. I took some time to set up the framed photos and other things I had brought to make the place feel more like home, but the knowledge that we would only be there for three months before having to find something else made it hard to completely settle in.

The next day, I called the Blackstone Walmart where I was going to be working and spoke to Rebecca, the front-end manager.

"Hi, this is Russ Dimino," I said. "I'm calling to get my hours."

"What do you mean, 'get your hours'?" she asked, already sounding annoyed.

"Oh," I said. "Um, I mean, to find out what my schedule is?" When I worked at Sam's Club, if you said you wanted to "get your hours," everyone knew you meant you wanted to know what hours you were scheduled for that week. Clearly I was going to have to get used to people saying things differently in Virginia.

"Well, you were supposed to be here last week," Rebecca snapped. "At this point I didn't think you were coming at all."

"Um, there must be some mistake," I said. "Last week I was still in New York. I was still working at Sam's Club last week. I'm supposed to start at your store this week."

"Well, I had you on the schedule last week and you weren't here," she insisted.

I was not sure what to say. Something had obviously been messed up with the paperwork. It wasn't my fault. After some more back-and-forth, she told me to come in the next day and I could start training. But the deck seemed stacked against me, and this woman now had a bad first impression of me before I even walked in the door.

I was not exactly thrilled to be working at Walmart. The feeling of being "stuck" at Sam's Club back home extended here. What I really wanted was to do something with film or television. My media arts degree from Fredonia was like a key, but I had no idea how to find the door that it went to. I thought of those TV stations and video production companies I had sent my resume to back home. I had given up hope on even hearing back from them by the time I made the decision to move to Virginia with Amanda.

I was about to find out that the universe either had a horrible sense of timing or a very strange sense of humor.

Chapter Three

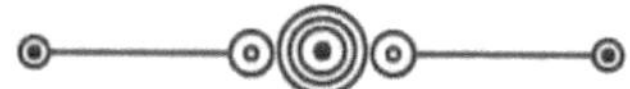

One day, out of the blue, I got a phone call from Craig, the production manager at 13 WHAM News in Rochester, New York. They were hiring for a part-time position in the production department, editing video for the news and operating the studio cameras during the live broadcasts, and he wanted me to come in for an interview. It sounded amazing. I would have absolutely jumped with excitement if I had still been living at home when I got that call. I reluctantly explained to Craig that I was no longer in the area and had just moved to Virginia.

When Amanda got home from work, I couldn't help but laugh as I told her about it.

"You're not going to believe this," I said. "I got a call today from 13 WHAM back in Rochester. They wanted me to come in for an interview!"

"Really?"

"Yeah! It figures, right?"

"What did you say?"

I shrugged. "I mean, I told them I just moved to Virginia, so I couldn't."

"You should do it," Amanda said, without hesitation.

"What?" I asked.

"Call him back and see if you can still get the interview," she insisted.

"But… we just moved here…"

"Russ, this could be the opportunity you've been looking for ever since we graduated. You can't just pass it up," she insisted. "At least go for the interview, meet them, learn more about it."

It was what I'd needed her to say without even knowing I needed her to say it. Honestly, it did not even occur to me to go for the interview because in my mind I had left Rochester behind. They might as well have called and said they had a job opening on the moon. But Amanda had a knack for knowing what I really needed even when I didn't know it myself. And she knew that I would kick myself if I didn't at least take that interview before making a decision about this job.

I hugged her as tightly as I could. Neither of us said it at that moment, but we both knew that if this job did work out, it would mean some difficult decisions for us. We weren't ready to have that conversation yet. One step at a time.

I called Craig back and asked if it was too late to schedule that interview, telling him that I would make the trip back home to Rochester for it. He was glad to hear that I'd changed my mind. We scheduled an interview, and I quickly made reservations for a flight back to New York.

As I sat at the gate waiting for my flight a few days later, I opened a small brown paper bag that Amanda had packed for me. Inside were eight cookies, each one with a frosted letter on it, spelling out the words GOOD LUCK. There was also a note telling me how proud she was of me and that she knew I would do great on the interview. I could not imagine a more caring and supportive girlfriend than Amanda. Even though there was an unspoken fact looming over this whole thing—that if I did get the job it could mean us being apart again—she was still rooting for me. That love and dedication was such a powerful thing that I sat there crying, reading and rereading her letter as I waited for my flight to board.

On a Thursday in December 2005, I interviewed with 13 WHAM News. The interview went great. The production manager was impressed with the demo DVD I had sent along with my resume all those months ago, which included some of my college projects and a short promotional video I had done for Mothers Against Drunk Driving. He was glad to see that I was a Fredonia graduate and mentioned that they had hired a lot of Fredonia grads over the years, and they were always great.

We talked about the position they were looking to fill, and he reiterated a lot of what we had talked about on the phone. It was a part-time position, about thirty hours a week, but it started out with a paid six-to-eight-week training program that was forty hours a week. The role would involve editing video for the news, operating the studio cameras for the live news broadcasts, and possibly going out on location for some shoots as well. It all sounded so fun and exciting.

As our interview wrapped up, Craig asked if I would like a tour of the station. Would I! It was approaching five p.m., so the evening news would be starting soon. We walked into the newsroom where the anchors and reporters and producers all had their desks. It was a bustle of energy and commotion. A producer was shouting out how many minutes were left until they were on the air. One of the editors raced past us with a stack of mini-DV tapes in his hand, headed for the control room. Another producer grabbed a stack of scripts off the printer and handed it to a director, saying there had been a few last-minute changes. It was a whirlwind of chaos that was both intimidating and exhilarating. Could I work in this madness every day? I kind of really freaking wanted to. Had they scheduled my interview at this time so I could see this? Probably.

We went up to sub-control next, which was where the director, AD (assistant director), sound board operator, and producer were making last-minute preparations. The director sat in front of a huge switchboard with dozens of buttons and faders on it that he would use to switch between cameras and video sources. On the wall in front of him were row upon row of monitor screens, showing a feed from each studio camera, another camera in the newsroom, a camera downtown that was set up for a reporter who was live on location, several different videos that were queued up and ready to play, a live feed from ABC, and more.

In the center was one big monitor that showed what was currently on the air. To the right of the director was a big window where you could look out over the studio as news anchors Doug

Emblidge and Ginny Ryan took their spots behind the anchor desk. Three big cameras surrounded the desk, each manned by a camera operator wearing headphones. There was a big green chroma-key wall a few feet away where the meteorologist would give the weather forecast.

As five p.m. hit, the AD pressed a button on a keyboard that rolled the opening clip. "This is 13 WHAM News at Five, with Doug Emblidge and Ginny Ryan," the voiceover proclaimed as theme music and animation graphics played. The director pulled one of the fader switches on the board as the animation ended, and the graphics on the big monitor faded away to reveal Doug and Ginny at the desk.

As the anchors calmly delivered the news that viewers saw on TV, sub-control was bursting with activity. The producer was talking to the reporter out on location, keeping her posted on when they would be taking her live shot. The director was talking on a headset to the camera operators in the studio, telling them what shot they needed next. The AD was pressing play on each video in turn just before the director cut to it. The sound-board operator was bringing the volume up or down on about a dozen different sources depending on who was talking or which video was playing. It was well-orchestrated, fast-paced mayhem that was somehow appearing seamless to the viewers at home.

My favorite part was near the end of one of the segments, which had been a humorous story about what to get a woman for Christmas. Doug and Ginny started ad-libbing and making jokes, going way off the script on their teleprompters. The producer was looking at the clock and freaking out. "Tell them to wrap it up!

Tell them to wrap it up!" The camera operators in the studio started making hand-waving motions to try to get the anchors to wrap. When they finally went to break, everyone had to regroup during the commercials and figure out which stories to drop from the next segment so that the show wouldn't run long.

As I was leaving, Craig told me that he was glad I decided to fly in for the interview. "I think you'll find it was worth your while," he said.

Back in Virginia, there was now a clock silently ticking in the background of everything that Amanda and I did. Not knowing how long we would have together there, we threw ourselves into celebrating the holiday season. We bought a Christmas tree, put up lights, and hung stockings by the fireplace. We would go out to the mall just to walk around, hand in hand, admiring the decorations and taking in the sights and sounds of the season. We cuddled on the couch and watched our favorite holiday movies like *Home Alone, A Christmas Story*, and *National Lampoon's Christmas Vacation*.

We opened presents on Christmas Eve. One of the gifts Amanda got me that year was a Billy Joel CD box set that included a lot of rare and unreleased tracks that I had never heard before. For a Billy Joel enthusiast like myself, this was quite a find, and I was very excited about it. I couldn't help but pop the CDs in on Christmas Day and start listening to them. One track in particular that I instantly fell in love with was a cover of "When You Wish Upon a Star." It was a very soulful, jazz-bluesy rendition of the classic Disney song. I looked at Amanda and I could tell by the look on her face that she was just as mesmerized by it as I was.

Without a word, I reached out my hand, and she gently put hers in mine. I pulled her close to me and wrapped my arms around her waist. We swayed back and forth in a sweet, spontaneous slow dance by the glowing light of the Christmas tree. For that moment, everything was perfect.

As 2005 came to a close, I had not heard anything back from 13 WHAM News. I chalked this up to the busy holiday season. Even so, I couldn't stop thinking about it. The job seemed so exciting. But I knew that taking it would mean leaving Amanda all by herself in Virginia after we had just moved down there together. How could I even consider doing that to her? My mind was a constant blur of enthusiasm tempered with guilt and regret. I constantly agonized over whether or not I should take a job that I hadn't even been offered yet. The uncertainty of it all was weighing on me.

Little did I know then that this ambiguity would be hanging over my head for the next year.

Chapter Four

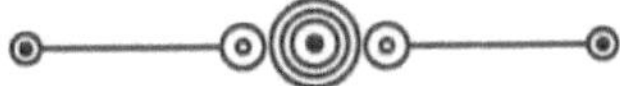

Our three months of free living at that big luxurious house on the hospital grounds had come to an end. Our new living situation was a real wake-up call, and only served to underscore how good we'd had it at the other place.

Amanda and I were now renting the first floor of a little house in Meherrin, which was about twenty minutes southwest of Burkeville where we had been before. When I tell you that this place was off the grid, I cannot emphasize this enough. The house was set back in a wooded area, and you could not see it from the street. It was so secluded that there was no garbage pick-up; you had to drive your garbage to the local dump yourself. No internet providers even offered service in that area. Even America Online's dial-up option was not available, as there were no local access numbers. We were about as far off the beaten path as you could get.

Also, while the previous house had been fully furnished, this place was not. We did not have much money to buy furniture, so we started out with lawn chairs as living room seating. The secluded nature of the house and the limited accommodations all added up to feeling like we were on the lam and hiding out at this joint.

The job at Walmart was going okay. My time was divided between running a cash register and manning the customer service desk. It was definitely a step down in responsibility from being a COS at Sam's Club, but I didn't mind. I was looking forward to having some anonymity here. I wanted to just blend into the background and go unnoticed. That did not quite work out. My Rochester accent made me stick out like a sore thumb any time I opened my mouth, which always prompted people to ask where I was from. I have noticed that anytime you say you are from New York to anyone who is not from New York state, they assume you mean New York City. Rochester is in western New York and is a very different beast from the Big Apple. It's actually pretty rural by comparison. But to my new coworkers, I was now the big-city boy who had moved out to the country.

I hadn't heard anything back from 13 WHAM after that great interview experience I'd had. After a couple of weeks, I gave Craig a call.

"We are currently under a hiring freeze here," he explained over the phone. "You're still in the running; we haven't filled the position yet. I just can't say for sure when we will be able to do so."

Through all of this, the symptoms that I described earlier continued to come and go. I was still assuming this was just some kind of long-lingering stomach bug that I couldn't completely shake for some reason. Eventually, I felt like I needed to do something about it.

I called my doctor back home in Rochester, since I didn't have one in Virginia yet. I explained that I was living out of state and had been having diarrhea on and off for several months, and I asked if there was anything he could recommend. As I said before, "diarrhea" wasn't really the right word for it, but I didn't know how else to describe it. He recommended that I try the over-the-counter drug Prilosec.

In 2006, on the two-year anniversary of the day that Amanda and I had started dating, I cooked a big chicken parmesan and spaghetti dinner to celebrate. We ate our anniversary dinner on a blanket on the floor of the living room, picnic style. The only problem was, it was my second day taking Prilosec, and I had absolutely no appetite. I had an anti-appetite. That feeling where the thought of eating anything seemed repulsive. I actually knew, even as I was cooking, that I wasn't going to be able to eat it. But it was our anniversary dinner, and I didn't want to spoil it by saying that I didn't feel well. So there we were, this big dinner and a couple of glasses of wine laid out in front of us, and I didn't feel like eating at all.

I managed to take a bite of chicken and chew it for about ten minutes. I'm not sure why I didn't think Amanda would notice this, but she did.

"Why aren't you eating?" she asked.

"What are you talking about? I am eating!"

"You're eating really slowly."

"It's so good, I just really want to savor it," I said.

"Russ." She had a way of saying my name that could instantly cut through my bullshit.

"Okay, fine," I said reluctantly. "My stomach doesn't feel good. It's felt lousy all day. I just have no appetite at all."

"Why did you still go to all this trouble, then?" she asked. "We could have postponed it and had it another night when you felt better."

"I know. I just wanted today to be special," I said. "I didn't want to ruin our anniversary."

But now I felt like I had ruined it after all.

The next afternoon, I went in to work for a closing shift at the customer service desk. I'd still been taking Prilosec and was waiting for it to solve all my problems. After all, it had been my experience that if you were sick, you went to your doctor, took what they recommended, and then you'd get better. I just figured it was taking a little longer to kick in.

That's when the diarrhea hit.

I've said a couple of times that I had been using the term "diarrhea" when it was not really accurate, but this, my friends, was straight out of the diarrhea textbook. The diarrhea dictionary definition. The prime example of diarrhea. It hit suddenly, coming in pure liquid form, and it made my bowels feel like a washcloth being wrung out.

The first time it hit, I was able to quickly excuse myself from the service desk and make it to the employee bathroom. When I emerged, I stopped by my locker. I had a box of Imodium in there because I was no stranger to having "emergencies" strike at work. I took two Imodium, which was usually enough to shut things down for a while.

Before I even made it all the way back up to the service desk, I had to turn around and sprint right back to the bathroom for round two. I sat on the toilet, guts exploding, trying to calm myself down. *Just give the Imodium time to work*, I told myself. *It will kick in any time and you'll be fine.*

I popped two more Imodium just to be safe. Four Imodium, I figured, was probably overkill, but it *had* to get everything stopped up to at least get me through my shift, right?

Wrong. Before I knew it, I was back in the bathroom for the third time in half an hour.

This was ridiculous. Something was really wrong here. I was used to having to deal with my sporadic stomach symptoms while on the clock, but I'd spent more time on the bowl than doing my job at this point, and there was no way I was going to be able to get through the rest of my shift like this. I needed to go home.

I found Joann, one of the front-end supervisors. She was a little older, a sweet lady, kind of a motherly figure who I figured would be understanding and have no issue with letting me leave. I told her I wasn't feeling well and needed to go home. She was sympathetic but told me I would need to check with the manager on duty for the evening, who happened to be Rebecca.

I didn't really relish the idea of asking her after the confusion we'd had about my start date. We didn't get off on the best foot, and even though it was clearly a misunderstanding I always got the feeling that she still thought of me as a slacker who blew off a week of work.

I swallowed my pride and went up to Rebecca and pled my case. I told her I didn't feel good and needed to go home. She immediately shook her head. "No way. We're short-staffed tonight. You're the only one working the service desk after Angela goes home at five."

I couldn't believe I was saying this next sentence out loud to my boss, but I had to convey the severity of the situation. I half-whispered through gritted teeth, "I have diarrhea." Yes, I said the word "diarrhea" out loud to my boss. It was a real career highlight.

"That's… too bad," she said, a little unsure of how to react to that statement. "But we need you here tonight. You know where the bathroom is. If you have to go, just go."

Well, there it was. I had to stay and work, but I had permission from my boss to use the bathroom if I needed to. Her sympathy and generosity will never be forgotten.

I went back to my locker one last time. I looked at the back of the box of Imodium. It said not to exceed eight tablets in a twenty-four-hour period. I'd already taken four tablets in about an hour and my ass still felt like a ticking time bomb. I popped two more and prayed that they would kick in soon.

The rest of the night went something like this: wait on a customer, run to the bathroom, repeat. There were times during the evening that I would walk away from the desk with a line of customers waiting to be helped, apologizing and assuring them I would be right back. All the Imodium that I had taken slowed things a bit but didn't shut it down.

Before my shift was over I took two more, hitting the maximum daily dose in a span of a few hours. It took me a very long time to realize something that you, dear reader, probably already figured out: the Prilosec was giving me diarrhea. Picture, if you will, a battleground in my large intestine where the Prilosec is opening some kind of giant floodgate, and the Imodium soldiers are rushing in with riot gear and trying to close it down but they are outnumbered because the Prilosec has been in there longer and established more of a stronghold and has the diarrhea floodgates very well defended.

By the end of the night I was completely exhausted. You know that worn-out, beat-down feeling you have after a nasty stomach bug? I had that, and I had just worked an eight-hour shift through it. As the store closed down and the last call for employee purchases was made before they turned off the registers, I grabbed a box of saltine crackers and a bottle of ginger ale. It was partly because I had that inherent craving for those items that comes with a stomach bug, and partly because I wanted to be like, "See, I really am sick, you bastards!" Joann rang me out and told me she hoped that I felt better soon. I could tell that she really did feel bad that they hadn't sent me home.

As we were all walking out to the parking lot to go home for the night, Jim, one of the other department managers, said to me, "Hey, do you drink a lot of beer?"

"Huh?"

"Do you drink a lot of beer?" he asked again.

"Uh, no, not really," I replied. "Why?"

"That can do that to you," he said. "Drinking a lot of beer can really mess up your stomach like that."

I nodded. "Oh. Okay," I replied. "Good to know."

So, Rebecca or Joann had obviously told Jim about my diarrhea, and he had taken it upon himself to give me the advice that maybe I was drinking too much beer. Awesome, thanks for the advice, dude.

I called in sick the next day. I stayed home with the comfort of my ginger ale and saltines. And guess what, I took at least one more dose of Prilosec before I figured out that's what was messing me up. Before you think I'm a total idiot, remember that this was the first time in my life a doctor had told me something that turned out to be wrong. It would not be the last.

I called my doctor in Rochester again and told him that things had gotten way worse since I started taking the Prilosec. He told me that this was beyond what he could help me with over the phone, and that I needed to see a gastroenterologist.

My health insurance came with a printed list of doctors that were "in network." This was my first experience managing something like this on my own. When I had lived at home with my parents, I was on their insurance, so navigating where I could go and what was or was not covered was all new to me. I looked through the list of gastroenterologists in my area that were in network and picked the one closest to me.

I called and made the soonest possible appointment.

Chapter Five

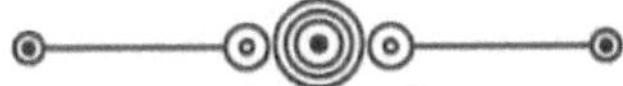

I got in to see this first doctor—I'll call him Dr. Harvey from here on—in Virginia in early March 2006. I told him about everything I had been experiencing so far. The urgent trips to the bathroom, the discomfort, the episode with the Prilosec, and so on. He said he wanted to perform a colonoscopy to see what was going on. We scheduled it for the following week, and he prescribed me some preparatory stuff to drink the day before that would "clean me out." Gross.

When I got home from the appointment, I called Mike back in Rochester. I remembered that he'd had some digestive issues when we were in college and had to go see a gastroenterologist, and that he'd had a colonoscopy as well.

"Yeah, man, the colonoscopy is nothing to worry about," Mike told me. "The worst part is the day before when you have to do the prep. It gives you the worst case of the shits you've ever had in your life." Mike was not one to mince words. "They dope you up so much for the actual procedure that you won't feel a thing. You come out of it feeling like you're in a tequila haze."

"What did they end up finding out from it?" I asked hesitantly.

"It was nothing serious at all," Mike replied. "I went in because I saw some blood in my shit and got really freaked out. But it wound up just being the fact that I was living on fast food and alcohol for the last few semesters, just like every other college kid. The doctor had me make some changes to my diet and I was feeling better in no time. I'm sure you're going to find out the same thing, buddy."

Talking to Mike made me feel a lot better. I also admired how honest and open he was about what he went through. He had just told me that he was shitting blood as casually as if we were talking about the Buffalo Bills game coming up on Sunday. The fact that it turned out to be nothing serious and he fixed it with some modifications to his diet was very promising. I had always paid such little regard to what I ate, I figured this was all going to turn out to be me just needing to be a little more health conscious.

As Mike had alluded to, the real pain in the ass (so to speak) with a colonoscopy was the prep the day before. I filled the prescription that Dr. Harvey had given me, and the pharmacist gave me this giant plastic jug that had some powder in it to mix with water to create the solution. It was called GoLYTELY, but trust me, it doesn't make you "go lightly." There are some other brands with their own variations on it called MoviPrep and some other ones, but they all achieve the same result. It also comes with some optional flavor packets that you can mix with it to make the stuff more palatable, in theory. Mine came with cherry, orange, pineapple, and lemon-lime.

The day before the procedure, I was to have nothing to eat or drink except for clear liquids in the morning. Then, in the afternoon, I added water to the big plastic jug and mixed it up to create the GoLYTELY solution. I added the cherry flavor packet. Then, at two p.m., I drank my first eight-ounce glass of the stuff.

I am not really sure what I was expecting the stuff to taste like. Maybe the cherry flavoring got my hopes up a little bit, letting me think it might be somewhat enjoyable. It tasted like what I would imagine dish soap tastes like, and with a similar consistency. Which I guess makes sense, as it's supposed to "clean you out," right? It felt like I was drinking something that would literally be scrubbing the fecal matter from my bowels.

Despite the unpleasant taste and consistency, it wasn't too bad to drink at first. I mean, it wasn't good or anything, but it's like taking medicine. You're not doing it for pleasure. You know you need to do it, so you just take it and get it over with. The instructions said to drink one eight-ounce glass every ten minutes until the stuff was gone. It was a four-liter jug, so that meant about sixteen glasses. That's a good chunk of time just drinking this stuff.

I tried to drink each glass pretty quickly. You could drink it slowly over the ten minutes, I suppose, but then you are pretty much doing nothing but drinking the stuff constantly, and I think that's worse. It seemed better to down it as fast as I could and then have as much "time off" as possible while I waited for the next round.

Amanda and I had just bought a new futon for the apartment so that we could retire the lawn chairs, and we figured since I was just going to be sitting around drinking the stuff and waiting for its effects, we could use the time to work on putting it together. This seemed like a good idea at the time. Neither one of us is especially skilled at assembling things, but we could follow instructions pretty well. We were a few steps in, and I had consumed a few glasses of the stuff and was not really feeling anything just yet. I wondered how long it would take before it kicked in. The directions that came with the GoLYTELY said it could take about an hour before the first loose stool occurred.

It was tough for me to tell, because I was used to always having to run to the bathroom at a moment's notice anyway. And drinking glass after glass of this stuff, you start to feel a little bloated, and you're not sure if you have to poop or if your stomach is just getting full of dish soap water.

I will tell you, though, that when it does hit you, it's pretty unmistakable. It is *your ass just turned into a water faucet* diarrhea. The one-hour mark is probably pretty accurate, but if you are ever doing this and it takes longer than that, I wouldn't worry. It will catch up to you sooner or later. It's going to work, trust me.

So here is the part that really sucks. You're drinking this stuff that, as I said, tastes like dish soap. It is giving you diarrhea. Like, really bad, sudden, forceful diarrhea. And you need to keep drinking the stuff. Ten minutes is up, down your next glass. Run to the bathroom. Sometimes you are in the bathroom for longer than ten minutes, so whenever you are able to get a moment of relief, you have to just get right to drinking the next glass. Repeat, repeat, repeat.

Meanwhile, your body and brain are having the natural reaction of, *This stuff is giving us diarrhea, we need to stop drinking it.* But despite your physical urge to stop ingesting it, you need to push that instinct aside and keep on chugging glass after glass. It's like in *Harry Potter and the Half-Blood Prince* when Dumbledore has to keep drinking the potion even though it's killing him. Maybe JK Rowling had just had a colonoscopy when she wrote that chapter?

Every physical inclination you have is to stop drinking the stuff that is making you sick, but you need to keep at it, and it is brutal. I had to just completely abandon Amanda to finish the futon assembly by herself, because drinking the stuff and pooping became a full-time affair. If you have to do this, clear your schedule for the rest of the day. This is really all you are going to be doing.

Even after I had choked down my last glass of the stuff, I found out it was the gift that kept on giving. The directions said "loose stools may continue for one to two hours after finishing the solution," but mine went on longer than that. Eventually it slowed down, but I would still have a sudden, smaller bout of diarrhea here and there for several hours, like aftershocks after an earthquake. I wished I'd started the prep earlier, to give myself plenty of time for everything to calm back down in my digestive tract. Honestly, the whole ordeal tired me out, and I wanted to get some sleep when I was done. The last thing I wanted was to be up all night as the last vestiges of the GoLYTELY finished their unholy work on my bowels.

I went to bed that night very worn out, but looking forward to the answers that the next day would hopefully bring.

On the date of my colonoscopy, Amanda and I arrived at the hospital early in the morning, with my procedure scheduled for 8:30 a.m. I was nervous, even though my conversation with Mike had assured me that the worst of the experience was the prep and that was now behind me (so to speak).

A nurse escorted us back to a pre-op waiting area. It was a small curtained-off room where I changed out of my clothes and into a very fashionable hospital gown. They gave me a bag to put my clothes in, and I gave my wallet and phone to Amanda. Then the nurse had me lie down on a gurney and checked my vitals, and she explained a little bit more about the procedure. They gave me a consent form to sign, being sure to explain all the possible complications and unforeseen events that could go wrong, including death, which sounded really scary, but if you think about it, couldn't something go wrong with pretty much anything you do that could result in death? I signed the consent form. Then the nurse hooked me up to a saline-lock IV, which went into my hand. This would be used to give me a sedative while they did the procedure.

I was so naïve about all of this that I thought the doctor was going to just pop in behind the curtain and do the colonoscopy in that little area. I was looking around and wondering what he was going to do it with since it was just me and the gurney and the IV pole. Did he carry the colonoscopy thing with him? Was it a portable device that he just pulled out of his pocket? I had no idea.

But it did make much more sense when they started to wheel my gurney out of that little curtain area and down the hall to a much bigger room that had a lot more equipment and such in it. It felt much more reassuring.

Once I was in the real room with the real medical equipment, they started giving me a sedative in my IV. And then… the next thing I was aware of was being wheeled back down the hallway to the recovery area. I was vaguely aware that time had passed, but I had not been cognizant of the actual procedure at all. I had that warm, hazy feeling you get when you partially wake up from a nap just long enough to realize you were napping, but you're so comfortable you just want to go right back to sleep. When people tell you the prep is the worst part of the colonoscopy, they really mean it, because you actually come out of the procedure feeling copacetic.

When I got to the recovery area, the nurse helped me roll onto my side. She told me I had to "pass the air" before I would be allowed to leave. For the colonoscopy, they blow air into your colon, like inflating a balloon, so they can get the camera in there better to maneuver around and take pictures. So before you can leave, you have to fart all that air back out. So, not only are you feeling all mellow and high on life from the sedative, but now you get to just sit there and cut the cheese.

After some time, Dr. Harvey came in. In a way I can't explain and still don't understand, he told me his findings so bluntly that it seemed like he was mad at me.

"You have inflammation in your colon and ulcers in your rectum and terminal ileum. For lack of a better term, you have

Crohn's disease," he said. "You will have trouble getting health insurance. You will have trouble getting life insurance. You will have a shorter lifespan." He then handed me three sheets of prescription paper. "This is a prescription for metronidazole, this is a prescription for ciprofloxacin. These are antibiotics. You will be on them for two weeks. This is a prescription for Pentasa. This is an anti-inflammatory. You will be on this for the rest of your life." Then he left the room without asking me if I had any questions.

I sat there stunned. My mind was in a completely unnatural state. On the one hand, I still felt dazed and relaxed from the sedative. On the other hand, I had just been given the worst news of my life.

This was not supposed to be the answer. Dr. Harvey was supposed to tell me a few changes to make to my diet. I would have to give up fried foods for a bit, I'd complain and probably make a few jokes about it to my friends, and I would be good as new in no time.

A shorter lifespan? At age twenty-three, you're immortal. The fact that you will die someday is so far off in the abstract distance that it's more like a remote possibility than a cold, hard eventuality. And yet I was just told that the hands on that doomsday clock had moved a whole bunch of ticks closer to my own personal midnight.

A doctor just told me that my own death was closer than I thought, and that I would be on medication for the rest of my life.

What the actual fuck.

Chapter Six

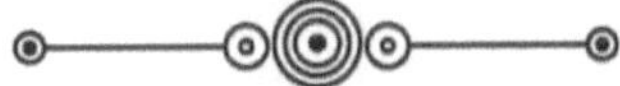

I took the prescriptions that Dr. Harvey had written for me to the pharmacy at the Walmart where I worked. I dropped them off before the start of my shift and picked them up on my lunch break.

"Picking up," I said to the girl behind the counter. "Last name is Dimino."

She went back and rifled through the small basket of bagged medicines marked "D."

"How do you spell it?"

"D-I-M..." I said. She looked through the basket a second time, seeming puzzled. "I dropped it off this morning," I said, trying to be helpful.

She looked at the computer screen. "Oh," she said, realizing why she couldn't find it. Then she went back and looked on the floor where there were several larger bags that did not fit in the little baskets. She came back with a big brown paper bag that looked like it could have held a to-go box from a diner meal you couldn't finish.

She scanned the barcode on the sticker affixed to the bag.

"That will be $212.20," she said.

I froze.

"Um…" I said slowly. "Do you need my insurance card, or…?"

"No, the insurance went through fine," she said. "That's $212.20 after the insurance."

Was this a mistake? What was I supposed to do? I wanted to say, "Oh, no thank you, never mind." Seriously though, did I *have* to get this? I didn't know. Even as I was still asking myself these questions, I handed the girl my debit card anyway.

When I got home from work, I showed Amanda my big bag of meds. Inside the bag were two small clear pill bottles—metronidazole and ciprofloxacin, the antibiotics—and two really big white bottles, which held the Pentasa.

"Can you believe this cost $212?" I exclaimed.

"Why did it cost so much?" Amanda asked, equally shocked.

"I don't know!" I took out the receipt. "I mean, at least this is the only time it will be that expensive! I don't have to refill the antibiotics, I'm only on them for a couple weeks."

I looked at the price breakdown for the first time. When I'd picked up the medicine, I'd been in too much of a hurry to stash it in my locker and get back to work.

The two antibiotics were $15 each. The Pentasa was $182.20.

I stared at the receipt in that mental state that you go into when you know you're screwed but your brain is still trying to make you believe for a minute that maybe you're not screwed. I don't know if it was denial or naïveté or a combination of the two, but up until that moment, I had really just thought, *Well, this is the only time I have to fill all three prescriptions, so from now on it will be cheaper.*

I would like to remind you again that I was twenty-three years old, living away from home for the first time, and just didn't have a concept that this was or could be reality. The fact that you could be prescribed a medicine that you needed to take on an ongoing basis that cost hundreds of dollars a month to fill… I mean, that happened when people got really rare debilitating illnesses or if they didn't have insurance. It couldn't happen to me.

"Amanda," I said. "Am I reading this right?" I handed her the receipt. "The Pentasa is the one Dr. Harvey said I have to take forever."

Amanda looked at the receipt. She looked at me.

"When's your follow-up appointment with Dr. Harvey?" she asked. "Could you ask him if you can take something else instead?"

"Yeah. Okay. That's a good idea," I said. "I have a follow-up with him in a few weeks, after I finish the antibiotics. I'll ask him if there's something else."

That settled it. That was easy. I would just ask him if I could take a different medicine. In the meantime, I'd start taking the antibiotics, and I'd probably see some improvement just from taking those.

Funny thing about antibiotics. Even though they help you get better, sometimes they make you feel a lot worse. It was just a couple of days after I started taking them that I noticed a funky taste in my mouth one afternoon. It was a gross, bitter, metallic taste that made me think back over what I'd eaten that day to try to figure out what could have left this unpleasantness behind. I brushed my teeth and tongue just to try to get rid of it, but it didn't work. It was like my tongue itself tasted that way. That evening, after I took another dose of my meds, the taste got worse.

Sure enough, as I looked at the list of possible side effects that came with the meds, metronidazole listed "unpleasant metallic taste." It also listed "nausea, vomiting, loss of appetite, stomach pain, diarrhea, constipation, rash, vaginal itching or discharge, mouth sores, or swollen, red, or 'hairy' tongue." I really hoped the metallic taste was the worst thing I'd get in my mouth and that I wouldn't end up with hair on my tongue. I was grateful that I didn't have a vagina.

I did, however, experience the diarrhea. It didn't occur right away, but as I continued the course of the antibiotics, it definitely showed up. At the risk of being repetitive, I will again point out that my usual day-to-day symptoms didn't really include what you'd consider "classic" diarrhea. Even though I'd take urgent trips to the bathroom, it wasn't the loose, watery stuff. The metronidazole, however, turned everything that was in my bowels into a soup-like consistency and hit the "eject" button frequently.

How cruelly ironic to treat a bathroom-related illness with medicine that gives you bathroom problems.

I suffered through the two-week run (no pun intended) of antibiotics defiantly, still confident that I was going to come out the other end of this (no pun intended… okay, actually, all the puns are intended) with this disease under control and living a better quality of life.

Dr. Harvey had also put me on a low-fiber, low-residue diet. This is common for people who have inflammatory bowel disease, as it cuts back on foods that are hard to digest and gives your intestines a little bit of a break.

Here are some things that are okay to eat on a low-fiber, low-residue diet:

- Refined or enriched white bread
- Plain crackers
- Cooked cereal like farina, cream of wheat, and grits
- Cold cereal like puffed rice and corn flakes
- White rice, noodles, and refined pasta
- Well-cooked vegetables without seeds, like green beans, carrots, mushrooms
- Cooked potatoes without skin
- Tomato sauce (no seeds)
- Ripe bananas
- Applesauce
- Eggs
- Lean meats such as beef, chicken, pork, fish

Here are some things to avoid on this diet:

- Skin and seeds of any fruits or vegetables
- Whole-grain breads, cereals, or crackers
- Raw vegetables
- Raw or dried fruits
- Beans, lentils, tofu
- Crunchy peanut butter
- Popcorn
- Fruit juices with pulp or seeds
- Tough meats with gristle

I had my follow-up appointment with Dr. Harvey a couple of weeks later. As I sat in the waiting room, a woman, probably in her late thirties or early forties, was at the checkout window, scheduling her next appointment. "Dr. Harvey is just the nicest man," she said to the receptionist. "Isn't he? Isn't he just the nicest man? He's so nice. He is just the nicest man." She said it so many times that the words "nicest man" started to sound funny.

I got called back to see the world's nicest man a few minutes later. We talked a bit more about my diagnosis. I remembered at the time of the procedure he had said, "For lack of a better term, you have Crohn's disease." He showed me some photos of my insides that were taken during the colonoscopy. You could see white blotches all over the place, which Dr. Harvey told me were ulcers throughout my terminal ileum, or the last part of the small intestine, and rectum. They had also taken a few biopsies and stool samples while they were digging around in there. In the biopsies of the terminal ileum, they noted granulomas and multinucleated giant cells. I didn't know what those words meant. I still kind of don't, but basically they found a specific kind of irritated, inflamed tissue. Dr. Harvey said that this was indicative of Crohn's.

He asked me how I'd been doing, how I'd been feeling, if my symptoms had improved. I said that even though I got a touch of diarrhea from the antibiotics, in general the meds and the low-fiber diet did seem to have calmed things down in my guts overall. I didn't feel like I was 100% again, but I felt more stable than I had in some time. He said he wanted me to continue the low-fiber diet for a couple more weeks, but that I was done with the antibiotics and to continue taking the Pentasa. He jotted down a few notes and started to leave without asking me if I had any questions.

"Well," I said quickly, trying to catch him before he was all the way out the door, "there is one more thing."

He stopped and looked up from his notepad.

"About the Pentasa. Even with my insurance, it cost me almost two hundred dollars to fill it," I said. "Is there anything else I could take instead?"

He seemed to be containing a sudden onset of anger. "I put you on Pentasa because you need to be on Pentasa. It's an aminosalicylic acid. It decreases inflammation. There is no generic version of it, which is why it's so expensive. In a few years, there probably will be one, but today, there isn't."

As he spoke, he walked over to a small cabinet and yanked it open. He reached in and started rooting around. "Insurance companies do not care if you live or if you die. They are in business to make money. They will cover you for what they have to, and nothing more." He grabbed a handful of pills in blister packs and pressed them into my hands. "This is Pentasa. This is what I prescribed you. This is what you need to take. Good luck to you."

And without another word he turned and walked away from me.

I looked down at the pills in my hands. They were blister packs of two pills each, which is a single dose of Pentasa. I had about a dozen of them. He had just handed me three days' worth of the medicine for free.

I don't know if he was mad that I questioned what he prescribed me, like I was questioning his judgement or something. Or if he was mad at the state of healthcare in this country. I am sure I wasn't the first patient struggling with affording their medication. But this guy had seemed legitimately annoyed when he gave me the diagnosis in the first place, and now he seemed downright indignant. Not fifteen minutes ago, that lady in the waiting room hadn't been able to stop talking about how nice he was. Was I seeing Dr. Jekyll?

I did not know it at the time, but this would be my last appointment with Dr. Harvey.

I did some reading up on the insurance coverage that I had, and why Pentasa cost so much. Pentasa was part of a classification of drugs called Preferred Brand Drugs. Like Dr. Harvey had said, there was no generic equivalent. They tended to be more expensive, and the insurance coverage that I had only covered 50% of the cost. In April, I sent a letter to my insurance company, asking them for additional coverage for my Pentasa. Here is the letter that I sent to Blue Cross and Blue Shield.

4/20/2006

To Whom It May Concern:

I am a Walmart employee, and I am covered under your CareMark plan. Recently I was diagnosed with Crohn's disease. My doctor prescribed me Pentasa 500 mg to be taken as two capsules four times a day. I filled this prescription at my local Walmart pharmacy on 3/13/06. Because this is a Preferred Brand Drug, my coverage only paid for 50% of the prescription, and I had to pay $182.20. I will need a refill soon, and this is more than I can afford to pay.

Because this medicine brand is medically necessary to treat my condition, I am writing a formal appeal for additional coverage on this medicine. I have enclosed my doctor's contact information as well. You may contact Doctor Harvey if medical information is needed for consideration of my appeal. Please inform me of any further steps I must take for you to process this request or any additional information you may require. I have also included with this letter a copy of the receipt for the medicine.

Sincerely,
Russell Dimino

I envisioned someone at the insurance company reading this letter and being moved by it. They would pass the letter around to their coworkers, calling everyone over to see it. The whole staff would be touched by my plea for help. "We gotta help this kid out," someone would say. There would be a genuine movement in the offices of Blue Cross and Blue Shield. My letter would be hung up on the bulletin board to remind each other of what they were really there to do. They would rally, they would pull the right strings with the right people, and they would increase my coverage for that one drug that I truly needed. Everything would work out in the end.

I never received a response to my letter.

Chapter Seven

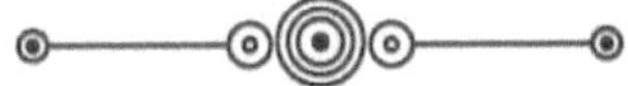

Our move to the new house meant a longer commute to work for me. It had taken me about thirty minutes to get from the Burkeville house to the Blackstone Walmart. Now my drive was nearly an hour, which was getting old fast. There was actually another Walmart that was closer to our new place in Meherrin, in a town called Farmville. (No, I am not making that up.) I put in a request to transfer to the Farmville Walmart, and Rebecca approved it immediately. I guess the fact that I had not made a great impression with her worked in my favor.

The Farmville Walmart was much bigger than the Blackstone one, and it was open twenty-four hours a day. It was a mere fifteen-minute commute for me, and best of all, it was a chance to start over yet again, with coworkers who were unaware of my diarrhea episode. Maybe I could do a better job of blending in here.

It was now September of 2006. One Tuesday evening, I was at home when I noticed a slight pain in my backside when I was walking or when I sat down. It wasn't really bad, but it was noticeable. Just a spot that felt a little tender. If I reached back and touched where it was sore, there was a small spot about the size of a pea that felt slightly hard under the surface of the skin and hurt to press on it. I didn't think much of it other than maybe I had pulled a muscle or something. I don't know how you pull a muscle in your butt, but it was the only thing I could think of. It didn't make much sense, but I figured it would go away in a day or two.

The next day, the spot still hurt, and on top of that I felt really tired and run down. I had to go to work, so I figured I'd just suck it up and deal with it. My energy level was extremely low. It was so bad that for my lunch hour, I went out to my car and lay down in the back seat and tried to get some sleep, setting the alarm on my watch to wake me up when it was time to go back in. I had no appetite, and I felt like I was maybe running a little bit of a fever as well. I figured I could tough it out for the day, but I just felt absolutely lousy.

At the end of the workday, I had to re-stack some boxes in the stockroom that had been put on layaway. It was a task that normally would have taken five, maybe ten minutes at the most. It took me about twenty that day. I was at the point where just walking across the room was a considerable effort, and now I had to rearrange giant boxes full of stuff. It was torture.

The next day, I was supposed to work again, but I just couldn't do it. I wasn't sure how I'd survived the day before, and the thought of going back in was not something I could muster. That little pain in my backside had gotten so bad that it hurt not only to walk, but to sit or lie down. Basically any position was painful.

I called in sick to work, with the resolve that if I still felt this way the next morning, I would go to the doctor.

Lo and behold, I felt even worse the next morning. The pain was spreading, and so was the hard spot on my butt. I called in sick for the second day in a row. I didn't have a primary care doctor yet in Virginia, but I knew there was a walk-in clinic in Crewe, which was about a twenty-minute drive from where we were living in Meherrin. Amanda was at work, so I drove myself to the medical center. It was extremely painful to sit all the way down on my bottom, so I used my left hand to steer, my right foot to work the pedals, and used my right hand and left foot to kind of raise my ass up off the seat. It was the longest twenty-minute drive of my life.

At the medical center, I saw a nurse practitioner named Michelle. I explained what was going on and where the pain was located, pointing to the area. I'd never seen a female doctor or practitioner before; I'd only ever seen male doctors. For some reason, I assumed she would not be able to examine my butt, like it would be inappropriate of her to do that or something. When she said to turn around and pull my pants down, I was almost like, "Wait, are you sure? Can you do that? Is this allowed?" Like it would somehow be unsuitable for her to look at my bare butt, even though that's precisely where my pain was located. It's not even that I was embarrassed or uncomfortable, I was just like, are we sure this is cool?

Michelle examined my buttocks and said that I had either a pilonidal cyst or a cellulitis infection. She prescribed me some antibiotics and some Percocet and said if it wasn't "dramatically improved" by Monday—this was a Friday—that we might have to schedule surgery to drain it. I started taking the meds and hoped for the best.

The Percocet helped with the pain, but not as much as I'd hoped. I was taking the maximum recommended dose of two pills every four hours. Within about ten to twenty minutes I'd be feeling great, but that would only last me until about the three-hour mark and the pain would start to come back. I'd be in agony by the time I hit four hours and could pop two more pills. I also had trouble urinating, I guess because of all the pressure building up down there. I'd feel like I had to go, and then I'd just stand at the toilet trying to get pee to come out and there would be just a trickle or nothing at all. I could not wait for Monday for my follow-up with Michelle. By Saturday night, it became so unbearable that I had Amanda drive me to the emergency room at Southside Community Hospital to have the cyst drained.

They removed fifty ccs of fluid from my cyst in the ER. They told me to expect it to continue to drain throughout the next day, and to see my doctor on Monday for a follow-up. The relief I felt was unbelievable. I was a little sore, but nothing like the pain I had been going through. I went from needing the Percocet constantly to not needing it at all. Plus, I could pee again! I had never been so excited to urinate in my life.

Before I left the ER, I told the attending physician I was concerned about all the time I was missing at my job.

"Could you write me a note for work?" I asked. "Something that just says I was at the hospital and why I was here?"

"They don't need to know why you were here," the physician replied with some concern. "They can't ask you that. It's none of their business. I can write you a note saying you were seen here, and that you should be excused from work for today and tomorrow."

This was news to me. I'd assumed that you needed to give your employer a good, specific reason why you had missed work, including what you were in the hospital for. HIPAA was not something I was familiar with yet.

The next day, I was puzzled. Nothing else drained out, even though they said it would. Then, gradually throughout the day, to my horror, the pain started to come back. I started having trouble peeing again. I reached back and touched where the cyst had been, and I could feel that area getting hard again. The cyst was filling back up.

I went back to the doctor's office on Monday and saw Michelle again. I explained I'd had the cyst drained Saturday night because of how bad it had gotten, but that now it seemed to be coming back. She examined me again and even brought in one of the other doctors to give an opinion as well. They both confirmed that the cyst was filling back up instead of draining out. They could see how much pain I was in, and the fact that the cyst had returned so quickly seemed worrisome to both of them.

Michelle walked me to the front desk and asked me to wait there a moment. She went behind the desk and made a phone call. She came back after a few moments and handed me a piece of paper, where she had written JOHNSON WILLIS HOSPITAL and the name of a doctor there.

"Do you know how to get to Johnson Willis Hospital?" she asked.

"No," I said.

She grabbed a large sticky note that had a logo for some medication at the bottom. She wrote the address and phone number of the hospital and the exact directions on how to get there. The directions weren't complicated, but it was maybe an hour or so away. Closer to Richmond, and a much bigger hospital than Southside Community where I'd had the cyst drained the other night. She handed the sticky note to me.

"Go there and ask for Dr. Bridges. He's expecting you and will see you today."

"Thank you," I said.

She nodded, and then said gently, "I'm sorry."

I will never forget the way she said that. It was genuine and sympathetic. I think it was partly her saying she felt bad for the amount of discomfort I was in, but also apologizing for not taking this more seriously the first time I came in and letting it play out over several days. I didn't blame her for that in any way. She made the best call that she could, based on what she saw.

But the fact that she made that call to the hospital, made sure I'd be able to see this new doctor ASAP, wrote out the directions to get there by hand, and apologized like that was a very personal gesture that has stayed with me for a long time. Or maybe we just had a special connection since she got to see my ass.

I called Amanda at work and told her what was going on and that they wanted me to go to Johnson Willis. Amanda worked about ten minutes away from the medical center I was at. I drove over to her work to meet her, once again supporting myself up off the seat with one hand and one foot, and she left work and drove me to the hospital.

Once we got there, I was actually surprised at how quickly I got in to see Dr. Bridges. From the time I checked in at the front desk to the time he called me back was not long at all. He and a nurse took me into an exam room and attempted to do the same thing they had done at Southside—drain the cyst with local anesthesia. I asked the doctor why it had filled back up and how we knew it would not do the same thing again. He said he wasn't sure, but that he was going to try to find out.

The doc drained the cyst again, but he wanted to make sure he'd gotten all of it, as he wasn't sure how deep it really went. Then, he found another pocket of infected pus deeper inside. I'm not sure exactly what he went in there with, but he had to dig inside me with some kind of instrument, going much farther than the anesthetic would numb. I can't begin to describe what that felt like. It was by far the worst pain I've ever experienced in my life. He was digging into a raw, infected cyst with cold, sharp metal and essentially no anesthetic due to how deep it was.

I screamed profanities that I had never said in front of strangers before. I didn't know what was coming out of my mouth. It was like I was not the one speaking. The sharp probe that was tearing and scraping my festering wound was also forcing out every swear word that had been buried in the darkest parts of my mind. It was like an exorcism of vulgarity. I gripped the table so hard my knuckles were white and just hoped and prayed that it would end immediately.

Finally, the doc stopped. The metal instrument that had just been inside my ass cheek clinked onto the tray like a fork hitting a dinner plate. "There's no way we can continue like this," he said, as if even he couldn't believe what had just happened. "It would be inhumane. We'll have to take you into the OR and sedate you."

Dr. Bridges left the room, and the nurse helped me get cleaned up.

"I'm sorry for swearing," I said, embarrassed by the string of obscenities that I'd screamed a few moments ago.

"No, honey," she said, shaking her head. "You were tough. I can't believe the amount of blood and pus that just came out of you." When a nurse tells you something like that, that's really insane, because you know she has seen some shit in her career.

Amanda and I were brought into a small consultation room with Dr. Bridges so he could quickly go over the details of the procedure we were about to do. He also said that I was one of the toughest patients he had ever seen based on what I just endured. I had a bottle of water with me because I was trying to stay hydrated. I took a sip of it, and Dr. Bridges promptly took the bottle right out of my hand.

"Um… you really shouldn't be drinking anything for two hours before the surgery," he said. It was a weird situation because we'd just decided a minute ago that I needed to go into surgery. We weren't about to wait two hours to do this, and it's not like we could go back in time and make it so I didn't drink anything. He handed the bottle of water to Amanda and said that the nurses would get me prepped.

I was officially admitted to the hospital and prepped for surgery. They were very fast and very efficient. The next thing I knew, I was in a hospital gown getting an IV stuck in me, sitting on a gurney, being told about how the procedure was going to go down.

An anesthesiologist had me sit at the edge of the gurney with my legs hanging over the edge and lean forward. He then stuck a small needle in my spine. It happened so fast and took effect so quickly I didn't feel any pain or even a poke, just a slight tap as if he tapped me with his finger. Then, I instantly felt a pins-and-needles sensation all the way down my legs, like when your foot falls asleep. They helped me lie back down on the gurney and then wheeled me into the operating room.

I was lying on my back with my feet up in stirrups. Dr. Bridges started working on draining the cyst again. It didn't hurt, but I could definitely feel that he was doing something.

"I can feel that," I said.

Dr. Bridges and the attending nurses all looked surprised. I don't think they expected me to be conscious, let alone remarking on what I could feel.

"I'll give you some more sedative," the anesthesiologist said, adjusting the IV I was hooked up to.

The next thing I remembered after that sentence was waking up in the recovery room with nurses checking my vitals as I stared up at the ceiling thinking how interesting the tile looked.

The scariest part was not knowing how long I would be in the hospital. I had assumed I would be going home that day, but the doctor said he wanted to keep me for a few days under observation to make sure the cyst wouldn't come back. This was understandable, and I sure as hell didn't want it to come back again either, but it was frightening not to know how many days I'd be confined to a hospital bed, and frustrating because I wanted so badly to just be home.

The next morning, Amanda walked into my hospital room with a Get Well Soon balloon and a little Ty teddy bear. She had taken the day off from work, even though she didn't have any sick days or vacation time available. I blinked away a few tears. No one had ever gotten me a Get Well Soon gift before. There had never been any occasion to. Amanda stayed right by my side all day.

I knew everyone back home was really worried about me. My mom was about two seconds away from getting on a plane and flying down, but there really was not much she would have been able to do if she had been there. We talked about it, and ultimately we decided that the money she would have spent on a plane ticket would be better spent helping me pay my hospital bills when I got out.

In the end, I was in the hospital from Monday until Thursday. The stay wasn't bad, but boy, was I ready to get out of there. The biggest headache was being hooked up to the IV all the time, so whenever I had to go to the bathroom I had to unplug the whole tower from the wall and wheel it behind me. Plus, if I wanted to take a shower, they had to come tape plastic over my arm where the IV tube went in so it wouldn't get wet.

They were giving me antibiotics through my IV as well, to keep the infection from coming back. On day two of my stay, I noticed a familiar, unpleasant metallic taste in my mouth. They were giving me that damn metronidazole again! Even getting it via an IV, it still gave me that funky taste in my mouth and made me feel nauseous.

Upon being discharged from the hospital, I was given a prescription to keep taking the metronidazole for another two weeks (much to my dismay), and they also told me to get a sitz bath. I didn't know what this was, but they told me that I could get one at any pharmacy. Basically, it's a little seat that you put on your toilet. It has a bag, almost like an IV bag, attached to it that you fill with water, and then it sprays the water up, all over your butt. Kind of like an on-the-go bidet. They told me to use this after each bowel movement to keep the incision area clean while it healed.

So, just to recap: I'm taking an antibiotic that actively gives me diarrhea, and also I have to take additional measures to keep this area extra clean. Amazing.

The sitz bath was actually kind of nice. I would fill it up with nice hot water, and it did at least feel pleasant to sit and have that spray up over that area. It took a little effort to set it up each time, though. I had to fill the bag up every time, and then find something to hang it on that was higher than the toilet. It took a good ten to fifteen minutes for the water to run through. So, as pleasant and relaxing as it was to use, I was going to the bathroom constantly and needed to do this after each time, so it was eating up a pretty big chunk of my day. Eventually I'd get bored and not even finish using it. I'd just let the water get about halfway through and be like, "Eh, that's gotta be good enough." It just got old after a while.

The diarrhea was way worse this time than the last time I was on metronidazole. I'm not sure if it was a higher dose or if my body had just developed whatever the opposite of a tolerance is to this medication, but it was giving me urgent, uncomfortable, cramp-your-stomach-up diarrhea. One time it even hit me so hard and so fast that I didn't make it to the toilet in time. I ran into the bathroom but ended up making a mess all over the bathroom floor. I sat on the toilet and started swearing, absolutely livid that I was having to go through this.

Amanda, who had heard me sprint to the bathroom and now heard me cursing to myself, came to the bathroom door to see if I was okay. She started to open the door to check on me, and I yelled, "Don't come in! Don't come in!" I didn't want her to see what had happened. I was so embarrassed. After I was done, I could barely hold back tears as I cleaned up the mess I'd made on the floor. Then I wearily filled up the sitz bath.

I didn't end up finishing the full course of the medicine. Even though I was worried that stopping it early might mean the infection would come back, I just couldn't put myself through the torture of finishing it. I stopped taking the metronidazole three days early.

Chapter Eight

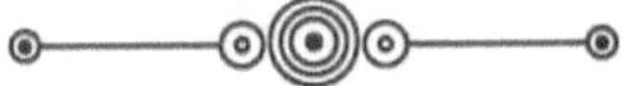

In October of 2006, I tried a new diet in an attempt to manage my Crohn's symptoms. My mom has always been the type of person where if you mention you're thinking of getting a new car, she will pull the last ten years of *Consumer Reports* for you and come back with a personalized list of what cars you should be shopping for.

So, knowing that her son had Crohn's disease, she was doing extensive research on how this disease could be managed. She mailed me a ton of stuff that she had printed out from the internet, along with a book she found that was written by a motivational speaker/health expert who had allegedly cured himself from Crohn's disease by adhering to a very specific diet.

I am not going to mention the book, the author, or the program outlined in the book by name. I am neither endorsing nor criticizing them. I don't want to create any undue implications regarding the advice in that book. It has many positive reviews on Amazon indicating that it was helpful to a lot of people. But it did not bring me the relief I was looking for, as I'll explain shortly. As such, I'm being intentionally vague about which diet this was, and I'll handle other books, programs, and diets similarly.

The first thing that you did on this diet was spend three days eating nothing but a special broth to give your guts some rest while still giving yourself the nutrients you need, simmered for over twelve hours. It cooks so long that the vegetables actually dissolve into the broth.

I will say this: from the very first spoonful, I could feel the restorative power of this stuff. Everything in it is good for you. It was comforting to eat. It just tasted healthy. However, eating nothing but the broth three meals a day for three days got old fast. I was so hungry that I was literally dreaming about food at night. Day three of the diet for me happened to fall on Halloween. I was at work at Walmart, and we were giving out candy. My coworkers kept trying to give me some, and I had to turn it down. No one I worked with knew about my Crohn's or that I was on this diet.

After the three days were up, I was able to add in some steamed vegetables and yogurt, but I also had to keep eating the broth. On day five, I went to eat some of the broth and I started gagging. I don't know if my body was just sick of it or maybe the batch had started to go bad. I started working on cooking up a fresh batch of it.

One day at work, I was heating up a bowl of the broth in the microwave, and one of my coworkers saw it and said, "Mmm! That smells so good! You got the right idea! I have to start bringing in stuff like that!"

Yeah, get Crohn's disease and go on an all-broth diet, it's awesome.

I had already been losing a lot of weight just due to being so sick. Now, on this diet, I was losing weight even faster. I was down to a mere 130 pounds, which was about fifty pounds less than I'd weighed before I got sick. I looked like I was auditioning for the role of Jack Skellington in *A Nightmare Before Christmas*.

One day at work, I started experiencing what I can only describe as butt leakage. Sorry, but there's no way to set some of these things up delicately. I didn't go to the bathroom or even feel like I had to, but suddenly I needed to wipe myself. It was like a faucet that was left on a little bit. It was really uncomfortable. It got so bad that I would take a whole bunch of toilet paper, wad it up, and stuff it into the back of my underwear to act like a barrier and hold me over until the next time I could get to a bathroom. Even so, every so often, maybe every twenty to thirty minutes, I'd need to run into the bathroom just to wipe and change out my makeshift toilet paper butt barricade.

At one point I was heading toward the bathroom when one of the managers waved me down. There was a customer with her who had a shopping cart full of groceries.

"Russ! Can you ring this customer up?" she asked. "She was waiting in line and we had to close down that register. It was acting up and we need to reboot it."

Now, obviously I wasn't going to say, "Hold on, I need to go wipe my leaky ass real quick and then I can help." I probably could have said I needed to go to the bathroom, but I didn't want to. I was too embarrassed to say that in front of a manager and a customer. So instead, I took the customer over to a nearby register and rang her up, clenching my cheeks together the whole time. All I could think about while I was scanning this lady's groceries was how badly I wanted to go into the bathroom and clean myself up, and how physically uncomfortable and just plain gross I felt. The very moment I handed that woman her receipt, before she even walked away, I sprint-waddled to the restroom to change my padding. Why was this my life?

In the fall of 2006, I had my annual performance review at Walmart. I was not a big fan of Darlene, the manager who gave me my review. She was not very personable. The phrase "resting bitch face" had not come into the public lexicon at that time, but if it had, it would have applied to her, although not only when she was resting. Most of my review was pretty good. I was always on time for my shift, always friendly, gave great customer service, and so on. Then she got to the last page of the review.

"The only issue is, you have a lot of unexcused absences," she said.

"I do?" I said, confused.

"Yes," she said. She showed me the last page of the review. It listed all the dates I had been absent. They were the dates that I had been out due to my cyst, many of which were when I was in the hospital.

"I submitted doctor's notes excusing me from work for all of those," I objected. "I was in the hospital."

Darlene just shrugged and shook her head. She didn't say anything.

"Why aren't those notes in my file?" I asked. "I gave them to HR."

"I don't know. It doesn't matter now, though. Once the review is written, we can't change it. An unexcused absence is an unexcused absence. There is nothing we can do."

I was livid. I had perfectly valid reasons why I could not be at work those days, and I had made sure to provide doctor's notes for all of them. Why would those be on my review as unexcused absences? And it's impossible to change the review after it's written? Says who? Are these reviews carved in stone? This was completely unfair. How did I know these "unexcused absences" wouldn't come back to bite me again later? What if I wound up in the hospital again? Were they going to eventually use this to fire me?

Darlene could tell I was mad. She just kept shrugging it off. "It doesn't matter," she said. "There's nothing we can do about it anyway. It really doesn't matter."

To her it didn't, but to me it sure did.

One day in October, my phone rang. It was a Rochester area code. I answered it.

"Hello?"

"Hello, this is Craig, the production manager at 13 WHAM News. Is this Russell?"

"Yes! Hi, how are you?"

"Good, good. I bet you thought you'd never hear from me, didn't you?"

I laughed. "Um, yeah, to be honest I was kind of starting to think so!"

"Well, as a matter of fact, corporate finally lifted our hiring freeze, and we're getting ready to fill that production spot that you interviewed for, it looks like it was a year ago?"

"Yes."

"Are you still interested?"

My heart skipped at least a few beats.

"Um. Possibly, yes. I'm still in Virginia right now. How soon are you looking to fill the position?"

"We'd be looking to have someone start next month, probably right before Thanksgiving."

My mind was racing. I needed to talk to Amanda. I couldn't make this decision without her.

"I am interested," I said. "But I need to talk to my girlfriend about this first. Can I give you a call back tomorrow and let you know?"

"Sure."

I was nervous to tell Amanda. It had been so long since the interview at this point that I really was starting to think that the job was just not in the cards, and we had moved past that specter looming over us. I went to Piedmont Hospital that afternoon to talk to her about it.

There was a thin layer of snow on the ground, which was rare for Virginia. Amanda and a group of her coworkers were outside, selling gumbo for a charity fundraiser. The sight of Amanda all bundled up in her winter gear to brace against the cold, ladling steaming hot gumbo into big to-go cups and handing them out to people with a big smile on her face stopped me dead in my tracks. She was such a sweet, kind person. She looked so happy.

"Hey!" she said, noticing me. Her grin grew even bigger. "Want some gumbo?"

"Oh, no thanks," I said. The hearty stew did look delicious on such a chilly day, but I had become extremely hesitant about introducing anything new to my volatile digestive system. "Hey, can I steal you for a second to talk about something?"

"Sure," she said. Her smile faded a bit, wondering what was up. She told her coworkers she would be right back.

We stepped away and walked out a bit onto the hospital grounds. Everything was so quiet and still in the cold, crisp air. The world around us was frozen in time. We were inside a snow globe, beautiful but fragile.

"What's on your mind?" she asked.

"I got a call from 13 WHAM News," I said hesitantly. "They're offering me that job."

"That's great!" Amanda said without missing a beat. She threw her arms around me in a big hug. "I'm so proud of you, honey. I know how excited you were about that job. You've been waiting so long to hear back from them!"

"You… are okay with me taking it?" I asked.

"You would be crazy not to," she said. "You'd finally be getting some real experience in your field. You have to do it."

We hugged again. Her unwavering support made me feel better and worse at the same time.

The next day, I called Craig and told him I would take the job, but that I'd need to give my current job two weeks' notice, and also make plans to move back to Rochester. We set my start date for November 20.

"One more thing," I asked. "The job is part time, right?"

"That's correct."

"Are there any benefits, like health insurance?" I asked. "Even if I have to pay more for it, is there any way I can get health insurance as a benefit being part time?"

"No, I'm afraid not," he said. "There are no benefits at the part-time level."

I was going to have to figure something out. Obviously I was not in any position to be able to go without health insurance now. I had my current insurance through Walmart. Walmart and Sam's Club do offer health insurance to part-time employees. The only way I could figure to make this work was to transfer back to the Sam's Club in Rochester, part time, work there on the weekends, and keep my health insurance through them. It felt like a long shot. Would they even take me back at all, let alone let me work only two days a week?

I called the Sam's Club in Rochester where I used to work and asked to speak to Julie, the HR manager who had helped me with my transfer to Virginia. To my dismay, I was told she was no longer working there.

My heart sank. The person who got me transferred out was not there to get me transferred back. Who could I even ask for that would help me?

"Um… what managers are working today?" I asked the woman on the phone.

"Coach Jerry is here… Coach Joe…. Coach Celia…" At Sam's Club, all the managers were called "coaches," like they were playing a ball game instead of working in a wholesale warehouse.

Coach Jerry was the store manager. He would have to approve my transfer anyway. Might as well go right to the top. I asked to speak to him.

"May I say who is calling?"

"Russ Dimino."

"Who?" Great. Whoever I was talking to had no idea who I was!

"My name is Russ Dimino, I used to work there."

"Okay." She put me on hold.

After a few minutes of hold music mixed with announcements about great Sam's Club deals, Jerry picked up the phone.

"Hello, this is Jerry."

"Hey, Jerry," I said. "It's Russ Dimino. How are you?" I hoped *he* remembered me. We had worked together a decent amount while I was there, but it had been a year…

"Hey, Russ, how are you?" he said. He either remembered me or at least was pretending he did.

"I'm doing good," I said. I'd better get right to my spiel. "Listen, I'm still in Virginia right now, but I got a job at 13 WHAM News in Rochester, so I'm going to be moving back. But it's only part time. I was wondering if I could transfer back to Sam's Club and work there part time too?"

"Sure, we'll take you back," he said.

I exhaled for the first time in ten minutes.

"Let me put you through to HR, and they can handle the details, okay?" he said. The guy was probably handling about twelve other things at the same time. He'd gotten on the phone long enough to give his verbal okay for me to transfer back, and that was all I needed. I talked to HR, and we hammered out the details of my new start date and such. I would be coming back as a cashier, because that was what they had available. At this point, I was grateful just to have a position to come back to.

The lease on the house we were renting would run out at the end of December. We knew I would be moving back to Rochester, and I wanted more than anything for Amanda to come with me. We had more than a few conversations about it.

"I'm not ready to leave yet," she said, apologetically but firmly. "I've only been at this job at Piedmont for a year. I feel like there is more for me to do here. I like where I'm working, I like my clients. I get to feel like I'm really helping people here and making a difference."

She made it clear that she would come back to Rochester, but when she was ready. And she was not ready yet.

"You're doing what you need to do," she said gently. "And so am I."

Most of the time, we were able to push the fact that I was leaving to the side and live each day like normal, as if nothing was changing. But not always. I could see on Amanda's face when it was starting to get hard for her, and I could always tell when she was thinking about it. "Hey," I'd say, taking her hand or stroking her cheek with my finger. "It's not time to be sad yet."

One night, as we were getting ready for bed, we were talking about my continuing Crohn's struggles and the fact that I still had not been able to get things under control, even after trying the diets and being on Pentasa for months now. With my move back to Rochester imminent, I casually remarked that maybe the move home would be good for me, and that maybe that was what I needed to really recuperate.

It was the absolute wrong thing to say.

Amanda burst into tears.

"What?" I asked. "What's wrong?"

"You don't think I'm taking good enough care of you," she said through her tears.

"Oh, Amanda…" I said. It felt like I'd physically inserted my foot into my mouth. I took her in my arms. "That's not what I meant at all."

"What else could you have meant?" she sobbed. "You just said you need to go back home to get better!"

"That's not…" I shook my head. "Honey, you have done an amazing job taking care of me. I could never ask for anyone more supportive and caring than you. I could not have made it as far as I have without you. It's killing me to leave you."

"Then why are you?" she asked.

In that moment, I didn't know. I truly didn't. All I knew was that my heart was breaking, and that the most important person in my life was in tears because of me.

"I won't go," I said. "If you don't want me to, I won't. I'll stay here with you."

She cried into my chest as I pressed my face against her head. What the hell was I doing? How could I leave this girl all alone?

Finally, she shook her head. "No," she said. "I don't want to keep you here. I can't be what holds you back."

It was gut-wrenching. Everything that had been left unsaid between us all of this time came pouring out in a flood of tears. We held each other, both sobbing, neither of us wanting to let the other go.

As it turned out, the day that I was to drive back to Rochester came on the same day that Amanda was going to fly to Kansas City for a music therapy conference. I made sure that I would still be able to drive her to the airport, and then I would just continue on from there. She helped me get my car packed with as much stuff as I could take.

Amanda had to fly out of Reagan National Airport in Washington, DC. It was a mess there. Somehow, every parking lot was full, even the economy lot. It was actually a good thing that I was driving her, because if Amanda had driven herself, I don't know what she would have done. I had been planning on walking

Amanda to the security checkpoint and seeing her off. Instead, I ended up dropping her off at the curb and leaving her to find her own way to the gate. I hated doing that, but in a way, it was for the best. It saved us from having a big, long, tearful goodbye in the airport. Knowing it was the last time we'd see each other for a while would have made it very hard.

Knowing that I would not be able to say everything that I wanted to when we went our separate ways, I wrote her a letter the night before. I thanked her for being so supportive of me, telling her how hard it had been to stay strong during these last few weeks when I knew I was leaving. I talked about all of those times I told her that it wasn't time to be sad yet, and how hard it was for me to do that. I didn't want her to think that I wasn't feeling the same feelings that she was. I was. I just didn't want us to sit around being depressed with the little time that we had left. I wanted us to enjoy every day, every moment that we still had together, and spend that time having fun.

Most of all, I told her that I loved her like crazy, and that I knew we would be able to do this long-distance thing, even though it would be hard. I knew there was no way that it would not work out, because we would not let that happen. We would not give up on what we had. I didn't want us to see the distance between us as an obstacle to overcome, but instead, as proof of how strong our love really was.

As we stood on the curb outside the airport, I gently put the letter into her hand and told her to read it after I was gone. She smiled and nodded, holding the letter close to her heart for a moment.

"I have something for you too," she said.

She reached into her bag and pulled out two mix CDs that she had burned for me. Written in marker on one was TO RUSS WITH LOVE. The other said RUSS'S ROAD-TRIPPIN' TUNES.

"Listen to these on your drive home," she said. "It'll be like I'm with you."

She always controlled the radio whenever we were on a long car ride together. Now she could still be my co-pilot, even though I was driving on without her.

I gave her a huge hug. "Thank you," I whispered into her ear, trying to keep my voice from breaking. "I love you so much, Amanda."

"I love you too," she whispered back.

We kissed. It was not the passionate, romantic kiss of two lovers who were about to be separated. It was a simple, gentle kiss, as if we were just leaving for a day of work. We knew we would see each other again.

Amanda grabbed her suitcase and wheeled it toward the airport door. I got back in my car and started driving north. I popped in the *To Russ with Love* CD.

"Time in a Bottle" by Jim Croce was the first song on the disc.

The hauntingly melancholy melody and lonely lyrics about not having enough time with the person you love, and how you wish you could save up every spare second just to share it with them, broke down any emotional walls that I had been able to keep up.

I could hardly see where I was going through my tears.

Chapter Nine

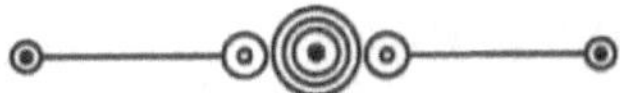

That uniquely Sam's Club smell of tires and baked goods took me back like an olfactory time warp as soon as I walked into the building. Many of the same people were still working there, but there were a lot of new faces too. The cashiers that worked at Sam's were an interesting mix. On the one hand, you had some who had been there forever, who had been working there long before I ever started and would probably be there long after I was gone. And then you had a very high turnover rate for the others. Kids just out of high school or working through college might be there for a summer, a semester, or a spring break, and then they were gone.

I was coming back almost exactly a year after I had left. One of the first familiar faces I saw when I came back in was the young, energetic front-end manager Coach Fred. "Russ is back!" he exclaimed. He came up and gave me a high-five, then walked me around to everyone, letting them know I had returned. "You don't understand! This guy is a legend!" he told the new cashiers. If only my Walmart managers had known I was a living legend!

Many of the familiar faces seemed really surprised to see me, but there was something more that I couldn't put my finger on. They were looking at me like they'd seen a ghost. Maybe they thought that me coming back meant that Amanda and I had broken up or something. Coach Fred's enthusiasm proclaiming my triumphant return and extolling my legendary status kept me from thinking about it too much at first.

I went to the breakroom to swipe my badge and clock in. One of the stock guys came up to me and said what everyone else seemed to be thinking.

"Russ! Welcome back, man. Hey, is everything okay?"

"Yeah, everything's fine! Why do you ask?"

"You just… you lost a ton of weight."

It had not even occurred to me because the weight loss had been gradual over the last year. But when these guys had last seen me, I was at least fifty pounds heavier. I looked gaunt. My face was skeletal. It was a dramatic difference. That's why everyone was looking at me so strangely.

What was I supposed to say? I didn't want to say that I had Crohn's. I didn't want anyone to know my secret.

"Yeah, I know. I'd been meaning to," I said, trying awkwardly to play it off like the weight loss was intentional, as if I'd just gone on a diet or something.

"But you didn't need to," he said, shaking his head.

I shrugged my shoulders. "Well," I said. "I thought I did."

It wasn't very convincing. At best, everyone would now think I was anorexic. I don't know that it was better than just telling the truth. But at the time, I didn't feel like I could tell anyone. I wanted everyone to think everything was normal. This was the first time I realized that, visually, it was actually very obvious that it was not.

The early days of working for 13 WHAM News were very exciting, even if they were physically exhausting. My shift was 3:30 a.m. to 12:30 p.m. The commute wasn't too bad, considering almost no one was on the road at that time, but it still took about half an hour. I'd set my alarm for 2:45 a.m., take a quick shower to wake myself up, throw on some clothes and drive in to work. I was usually one of three production assistants on that early-morning shift.

The producer of the morning show and the anchors would write scripts for the news stories and then tell us where to find the raw video to go along with each one. If it was a local story, it would be footage that one of the station's photographers shot. If it was a national news story, it would be from the Associated Press or another news outlet. We would take the raw video and edit it down to about thirty seconds to run as a "VO," which was a clip that the anchor would "voice over." Other times we would need to grab a sound bite from an interview to run as part of a story. That was called an "SOT" or "sound on tape."

We would head into the studio just before five a.m., which was when the live broadcast started each day. The three of us would operate the big studio cameras. We wore headsets; the director, in sub-control, would call out which anchor was going to read the next story and which camera to point them to. It was all very exhilarating and fun to be a part of, especially in those early days. The novelty of it all made it worth getting up so early.

We were on the air from five a.m. to seven a.m. straight. Then, from seven a.m. to nine a.m., we just did what were called "cut-ins" every half an hour, where we would be back on live for just a few minutes at the top and bottom of the hour to do a couple of quick top stories and the weather forecast. In between each cut-in, we got to sit around and watch TV in the editing bays.

Then, at nine a.m., we had an hour lunch break. We'd come back at ten and start getting ready for the twelve p.m. news. Same process as the morning—we'd edit video footage for the noon show, and then run camera in the studio. The twelve p.m. news was only half an hour, so after the two-hour morning show, it felt like a breeze. I was done for the day at 12:30 p.m.

Some days I would go home and take a nap. Other days I would try to power on through. I tried to stay on a routine of going to bed early during the week. I'd be in bed by 7:00 or 7:30 p.m., but even though I was bushed it was often hard to fall asleep at that time.

On the weekends, I worked at Sam's Club. My hours varied, but usually I'd be working eight-hour shifts both days, or sometimes an eight-hour shift one day and a five-and-a-half-hour shift the other. Working seven days a week was brutal, but the fact that the jobs were so different helped to break up the week and provide some variety, so it didn't feel quite so nonstop. Plus, I was only going to be working these five-day, forty-hour workweeks at

13 WHAM for my first six weeks while I was in training. Then, my schedule there would slow down. In theory.

It was hard being away from Amanda. I felt guilty, like I had abandoned her. She had moved out of the house we had been staying in and into an apartment with a girl named Audra, so at least she wasn't stuck in the middle of nowhere anymore. We'd talk on the phone at night, but by the time she was home from work and able to talk, I was exhausted. I'd usually lie in bed while talking to her, and by the end of the conversation I'd be struggling not to doze off. She would ask when I was coming back down to Virginia to visit. I wanted to so badly, but I also wanted to make a good impression at 13 WHAM, and I didn't feel like I could ask for time off so soon.

The alarm clock going off at 2:45 a.m. was absolutely brutal. My body did not get used to waking up at that time, no matter how many times I did it. It just wasn't natural. I'd hear the alarm, and it was like every molecule in my body was saying, *No fucking way*. The blood in my veins felt cold, like my heart hadn't had a chance to warm up yet.

Of course, during all of this, my biggest concern was access to the bathroom when I needed it. At 13 WHAM, I had three options. There was a men's room with two stalls and a couple of urinals right outside the recording studio; a large single-occupant restroom near the receptionist's desk at the front of the building; and a very small, almost closet-sized single-occupant restroom outside of sub-control.

My favorite one to use was the one near the front of the building, since it was big and it was just generally a nicer restroom. Because of its location, it was the one that visitors to the station would be most likely to use. Since it was just for one person and had a lock on the door, I had the most privacy in that one. However, it was a farther walk to get to that bathroom from the edit bays or the studio. If I was in a hurry, I might not have time to go to that one. And if I went all the way to that one and the door was locked because someone was already in there, I'd just wasted valuable time going out of my way. I could really only use it if I had time to spare, like when I was on a break or if we had a lull in editing and were not going on the air anytime soon.

The one right outside the studio I could get to pretty quickly most of the time, but I hated that there was limited privacy in there, and people were always coming in and out. I could get to the one outside sub-control quickly as well, but again, if it was locked, then I had wasted valuable time, and the pit crew—the team that tuned in the satellite feeds and ran some of the other tape decks and encoders while we were on the air—could see when anyone was going in and out of there. I didn't really want them to see me hurrying in and out of that restroom too often.

At Sam's Club, there were three bathroom options as well. The public men's room, a wheelchair accessible single-occupant bathroom, and a single-occupant restroom off of the employee breakroom. My preferred bathroom was the public men's room. Yes, it had a lot of people coming and going at all times, but it was different because it was mostly a lot of customers and not just my coworkers. Much less likely for someone to be like, "Wait, Russ is in here again?"

I liked the privacy of the handicapped bathroom, but I always felt worried that maybe someone in a wheelchair would need it and I'd be in there, or that someone would judge me if they saw me coming out of it. My absolute last resort was the employee bathroom, unless it was at a time when no one was in the breakroom, because everyone in the breakroom could obviously see you going in or out of that one. Also, it wasn't as soundproof as you might think a breakroom bathroom ought to be.

Those days, I was getting my Pentasa prescription filled at the Sam's Club pharmacy because it seemed super convenient. After all, I was there two days out of every week anyway. But what I didn't realize at first was the Sam's Club pharmacy was closed on Sundays. So now there was only one day a week that I was there. And the pharmacy closed for an hour at noon every day for lunch. If I needed more Pentasa, I had to try to make sure I got it on Saturday, and I had to make sure I took my break or lunch at a time when the pharmacy was open and not too busy. Sometimes I could pick it up at the end of my shift, but that was only an option if I wasn't working right up to closing time, which I often was.

But the timing of when to pick up my meds wasn't the worst part. My Pentasa refill came in two big bottles of pills, which they would put into a large brown bag and staple shut. The bag was so big that they couldn't fit it in the little bins on the shelf; it would be on the floor, just like it was the first time I picked it up at Walmart. It was huge and conspicuous.

Whenever you were leaving, they would have an exit door greeter check your purchases and your receipt, and this included employees. With pharmacy items, they weren't allowed to do that because of HIPAA, but there was always still an awkward moment when I was about to go out the door, when the exit greeter would anticipate looking at my receipt, and I'd have to hold up my giant-ass brown bag and say, "This is from the pharmacy." The exit door greeter would look surprised that I was picking up a grocery-bag-sized item from the pharmacy, but they'd let me pass without further inspection. I'm certain that this did not do anything to lessen the speculation around the club that something was wrong with me.

Christmas rolled around. Amanda took a week off of work and came up to Rochester to visit for the holidays. It had only been about a month since we had last seen each other, but considering we used to be together every single day, it felt like much longer.

Amanda stayed at her parents' house in Middleport, which was about forty-five minutes away from where I was living with my parents. For the week that she was in town, I visited her every single day after work, eschewing my early bedtime and hanging out well into the evening. I just couldn't bring myself to call it an early night when I knew that our time together was so limited. I would stay at her house until almost nine p.m., get home and be in bed by ten, only to get up for work at 2:45 a.m. I should've been dead tired, but I wasn't. Each morning the alarm would go off, and my first thought was that I would get to see Amanda again after work. It energized me. Being with her made everything brighter.

At the end of the week, saying goodbye again was even harder than it had been when I left Virginia. We'd had a taste of being together again after a month of phone calls and computer screens.

"When can you come visit me?" she asked.

"Soon," I said. "My training at the station is wrapping up. My work schedule should calm down after that."

As those initial six weeks of training at 13 WHAM came to an end, I was looking forward to being able to take my foot off the gas. At the end of week six, Craig called me into his office to talk about how things had been going.

"It's going great!" I said. "It's really exciting. Everyone's been super nice and helpful. I'm learning a lot." I truly was having fun and really liked working there, despite the insanely early hours.

"Glad to hear it," Craig said. "I'm working on the schedule for the next few weeks now. I'd like to get you working some weekends."

"Oh," I said. "I'm not sure how that's going to work. I have another job at Sam's Club that I work just on the weekends." I hadn't really thought about this. I knew that the six weeks of training was Monday through Friday, but I hadn't considered that they'd want me to work on the weekends after that was over.

"Well, do you think that's something that you could change?"

"Yeah, sure," I said, nodding and trying to sound like this wasn't stressing me out. "Yeah, I'll check and I'll let you know."

As I left Craig's office, I tried to think of how this would even work. I loved my job at 13 WHAM, but I *needed* the job at Sam's Club because that's how I was getting my health insurance. I felt like I'd gotten really lucky in that they took me back when I transferred from Virginia and let me come back only working two days a week. Saturday and Sunday were the busiest days at Sam's. If I asked if I could stay two days a week but switch them to weekdays, I felt like I'd be pushing my luck. There was no way they'd need me for just two weekdays. And would it always be the same two weekdays every week, or would it be random all the time? The thought of trying to juggle two work schedules that would be different week to week was a logistical nightmare. There was no way I could manage it.

Instead of going back and talking to Craig again in person, I took the easy way out and sent him an email. I said that Sam's Club only needed me on the weekends and that they couldn't accommodate moving my schedule to weekdays. I didn't know if he would be mad about it, but I had to trust that he wouldn't fire me after spending six weeks training me. I felt like I had a lot more to lose if I made myself less valuable to Sam's Club by saying I couldn't work weekends than I did by telling WHAM I couldn't work weekends.

When my first post-training schedule went up at WHAM, I saw that I was still on Monday through Friday, but on shorter shifts. 3:30 a.m. to 9:00 a.m. So I'd still be working seven days a week, and I'd still be getting up at 2:45 a.m. five days a week. Not even close to the respite I'd been counting on.

How long could I keep this up?

Chapter Ten

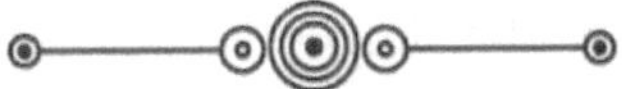

Now that I was back in Rochester, I needed to find a new gastroenterologist. I wasn't too broken up about having to leave Dr. Harvey, given his bipolar bedside manner. Maybe a new doctor would be a bit more sympathetic, or at least more consistent. I called my old primary care doctor—the one from the Prilosec debacle—and asked if he could refer me to a GI doc in the area. He recommended Dr. Griswold. There was a bit of wait to get in to see him. My first appointment with him was in March 2007.

Dr. Griswold entered the room, and it was like he was ready to do a comedy act. He had a notepad, and he reached into his breast pocket for a pen but pulled out a rectal thermometer instead. "A thermometer?" he exclaimed. "That means some asshole's got my pen!"

The joke definitely put me at ease, along with Dr. Griswold's laid-back manner. He sat and talked with me for a lot longer than Dr. Harvey had. He told me about the history of Crohn's disease, that it was discovered in the 1930s, that it was named after gastroenterologist Dr. Burrill Crohn, one of the doctors who first defined the disease. Dr. Griswold said that there was no cure for Crohn's disease yet, but that's because we were still learning about what causes it, and that he felt there probably would be a cure for it in my lifetime.

He talked about the importance of chronic suppressive therapy to keep the inflammation down. He told me to continue on Pentasa since I seemed to be generally well maintained on it, and he added a Cortenema for me to take for three or four weeks. He also sent me for bloodwork so he could check my CBC levels. I felt comfortable with Dr. Griswold, and I left my first appointment with him feeling optimistic overall.

Around this time, a new opportunity presented itself at Sam's Club. One of the managers, Coach Bob, approached me to give me a heads-up about an available position.

"Mister Russ," he said. He always called me that. "We've got a spot opening up in the cash office. I was wondering if you'd be interested in it. We need someone who is reliable and trustworthy, and you fit that bill. You'd have to apply for it and interview for it, of course, but I thought I'd put a bug in your ear in case you're interested."

It meant a lot to me to know that even after leaving and coming back, I'd still made a memorable impression, and that it was one of honesty and integrity. Working in the cash office— also called the accounting office or the business office, depending on who you were talking to—was no joke. You were in a small room with potentially tens of thousands of dollars in cash at times. Obviously they couldn't put just anyone in there.

The idea of any change of pace sounded great to me, and being able to get away from standing at a cash register all day was appealing. I couldn't help but wonder if this would make getaways to the bathroom easier or harder. I hated that this had to be part of the equation, but sadly it was one of the first things that came to mind.

"I would definitely be interested," I said. "Um, you know I'm just working weekends right now, though, right? Are they really looking for someone to just work two days a week?" I wanted to make sure my limited availability wasn't going to take me out of the running.

"I don't think that would be a problem," Coach Bob said. He suddenly got very serious. "I have a question for you, though. Are you claustrophobic? Could you handle being in a very small room for long periods of time? Because sometimes people freak out. We've had people run out of the room in a panic before because they couldn't take it."

"Oh. Um, I don't think that would be a problem…" I said.

I ended up getting the job. Most of the other associates who worked in the office weren't crazy about working weekends anyway, so having me taking some of those shifts was not frowned upon.

On my first day working in the office, I was training with a girl named Kelly. "Did Coach Bob ask you if being in a small room would freak you out?"

"Yes!" I said.

She rolled her eyes. "He always asks everyone that. No one has ever run out of this room screaming. I don't know why he tells everyone that."

The opening shift in the business office involved a lot of paperwork and filling out reports from the previous day. It wasn't hard, but it was time-consuming. A lot of the reports were printed on a dot matrix printer hooked up to what I'm sure was one of the first computers ever made.

On a good day, the print job ran automatically, and when you came in for the morning shift, there was a continuous form printout the length of two football fields waiting for you. On a bad day, the printer messed up and got jammed, and the first order of business for the day was unjamming this antique printer and navigating through two dozen DOS prompts to get it to re-print, then waiting an hour for it to print everything back out. There were more bad days than good.

But other than the unpredictability of the printer, the morning shift was not a bad gig. It was quiet, I was in an office by myself, there was a radio in there that I could turn on if I wanted to, and no one generally bothered me.

Meanwhile, some changes were also happening at 13 WHAM. The station was Rochester's local ABC affiliate but had recently acquired the local CW affiliate as well. With two channels to broadcast content on, the decision was made to expand the morning news programming. Now we would air four straight hours of morning news. Five a.m. to seven a.m. on channel 13

(ABC), and seven a.m. to nine a.m. on the CW. Gone were the days of having a couple hours of downtime to watch TV in the edit bays in between the cut-ins. Being on the air for four hours meant we needed production crew in the studio for four hours.

However, since we would also have new stories for those second two hours, we needed one person in the edit bays to continue editing and attaching video. We still only had three production assistants working that early-morning shift, which meant two people going into the studio at five a.m. One person would operate one camera, and the other would hop back and forth between the other two cameras. The third member of the morning crew would stay back in the edit bays and keep working on video for the CW show.

Now, you might be saying to yourself, "Wow, Russ, that sounds perfect! You could stay back in the edit bays and have more flexibility to use the restroom when you need to!" You would be very reasonable in thinking this. However, this would require me speaking up and saying that I would like to be the one to do that. I rarely did so. Even though being in the studio was much more difficult and anxiety-provoking for me, because being live on air severely limited how often I could run to the bathroom, I never voiced this to anyone. Being the "new guy" on the team, I didn't feel like I had the right to say I would prefer to stay back in the edit bays. It was definitely seen as the preferable role to everyone, as it was less physically demanding than being on your feet operating a big clunky camera for hours on end.

I could have said, "I have Crohn's disease, and working in the edit bays is a reasonable accommodation for my disability," but as you may have surmised from everything you have read up to this point, I was not going to do that. None of my coworkers knew that I had Crohn's, and I wanted to keep it that way.

As it turned out, we would typically rotate who went into the studio and who stayed back to edit, and I ended up editing about one day a week. I would look forward to that day so much because it was infinitely less stressful for me. I was so thankful just to be able to run to the bathroom anytime I needed to. Again, to be perfectly clear, no one knew I needed that accommodation because I did not speak up about it.

With the addition of two more hours of content every morning came the addition of a new morning show anchor. Evan Dawson, who had already been part of the 13 WHAM News staff as a reporter, now joined the anchor desk for those second two hours on the CW. After the announcement was made, Evan invited everyone from the morning show crew out for dinner and drinks.

We went out to a restaurant in downtown Rochester that did wood-fired pizza. I was excited to be out with everyone. I had been slow to make work friends since I was always so quiet; I preferred to remain in the background as much as possible. I was usually running on fumes at work and trying to hide how horrible I felt. The idea of being out with everyone in a social setting seemed fun though. I just hoped I could get through it without getting sick. I ordered the "plainest" thing on the menu, a small pizza with just cheese.

It ended up being a great time, with all of us talking and joking around for hours. At one point Evan suggested we go around the table and all share the last movie that made us cry. He said his was *My Life,* the Michael Keaton movie about a dying man who records a video journal for his unborn son.

"Mine is embarrassing," I said when it was my turn. "But it's *Armageddon.* At the end, when Bruce Willis stays behind on the asteroid so that Ben Affleck can go home and marry Liv Tyler."

"Russ, you're absolutely right," Evan said earnestly. He paused for a beat, then said, "That is embarrassing!"

We all burst out laughing. It was a great moment. I felt connected to everyone. Was I starting to fit in and actually belong? I hadn't felt like this in a long time.

On the drive home, I started to feel that all-too-familiar tension in my stomach. The heaviness, the pressure. I knew I was going to have to go to the bathroom imminently. It felt like a re-creation of that commute to Sam's Club, back when this all started, as I used every ounce of willpower I could muster to hold it all in.

It wasn't enough.

As I pulled into my parents' driveway, I shit my pants.

It was like the penance I had to pay for going out, having fun, and eating food. My Crohn's disease felt like a demon that was taunting me. A sinister phantom looming over me, chiding me for having the gall to think I could actually lead a normal life. As I sat in my own soiled pants in the driver's seat of my car in the driveway, I felt like maybe I didn't deserve to have fun.

I felt so alone.

One morning, as I was wrapping up my shift at 13 WHAM, I saw that I had missed a call from Amanda. It was unusual for her to call me so early in the day. I hoped everything was all right. I called her back right away.

"Hey!" I could hear the smile in her voice when she answered. It made me smile too.

"Hey!" I said. "I saw I missed a call from you. What's up?"

"I wanted to let you know that I'm going to be in Rochester next week!" she said.

"That's awesome!" I said. "What's the occasion?"

"Oh, nothing much," she said coyly. "Just a job interview!"

Amanda had gotten a call from her friend Lauren who was a music therapist at Heritage Christian Services in Rochester, letting her know that Heritage was looking to hire another full-time music therapist. Amanda had applied for the job without telling me. I think she didn't want to get my hopes up about the idea of her moving back. But when she got the call to come in for an interview, she couldn't keep it a secret any longer. I was excited just to be seeing her again when she came into town for the interview in April. I tried not to think about the fact that we might finally be able to be together again every single day if she got the job.

I saw Amanda after her interview. We got dressed up and went out to a nice Italian restaurant. I was always so nervous and paranoid any time I went out to eat. I had given up the all-broth diet, but I was still so cautious and careful about everything I ate. I tended to stick to a very bland diet most of the time. Have you ever heard of the BRAT diet? It stands for Bananas, Rice, Applesauce, Toast. It's most commonly used for little kids who have a stomach bug because they are easy to tolerate. These had become staples in my own diet for the same reason. Going out to eat at a restaurant where I had limited control over the ingredients in the food or how it was prepared was like rolling the dice. But with Amanda sitting across from me, candlelight dancing in her blue-green eyes, soft music playing, and the prospect of us being reunited again soon, I was able to back-burner my culinary concerns for one night.

Amanda had not been back in Virginia long at all when she got the phone call from Heritage offering her the job. She accepted it. In order to ensure adequate time to transition her caseload at Piedmont to her replacement and make plans to move back from Virginia to New York, she was able to set her start date for four weeks out. Meanwhile, I was like a kid counting down the days until Christmas. I had a crucial mission to carry out during those four weeks—finding somewhere for us to live.

I began apartment hunting right away. My mom came with me to every place I checked out. One thing that I was not willing to compromise on: it had to have more than one bathroom. There had been enough times when we were living in the Meherrin house in Virginia when Amanda was in the bathroom and suddenly I had to go. Any time she would even go to take a shower, it would stress me out not knowing when I could get in there if I needed it. Two bathrooms was a necessity in my mind.

But that seriously limited our options. Many apartments, even two-bedroom ones, still only had a single bathroom. There were other factors to consider, of course. The commute to our jobs. The rent. Whether or not utilities were included. What kind of neighborhood it was in. It was hard for me to keep all of these other factors in mind when the real litmus test for me was the bathroom situation.

After much searching and ruling out many locations that did not fit the bill, I finally found just the right place. Chili Heights Apartments had a two-bedroom, one-and-a-half bath available. The commute to 13 WHAM for me and Heritage for Amanda would be about fifteen minutes tops, probably less for me in the wee hours of the morning. Sam's Club on the weekends would be nearly as close, just in the opposite direction. The unit we would be in was a short walk from the complex's main office building, laundry room, swimming pool, and tennis court. I couldn't see myself using those last two amenities too often, but it was still nice to have them.

As I stood in the empty unit looking around, the bare white walls seemed like blank pages to me; their emptiness symbolized the potential to start a new chapter. It was about to be me and Amanda together again, ready to face the world, only this time much closer to home.

We did things right this time and actually got some furniture. No more lawn chairs or blankets on the floor. We hung framed photos on the walls. Unlike the temporary housing at Piedmont Hospital or the first floor of that secluded house in Meherrin, this felt like ours. A place where we could settle in and get comfortable. It felt like the new season of a favorite TV series about to start, but the writers had made some changes, brought back some beloved characters, and put our heroes in a new setting.

Now if only we could get those hacks to wrap up this damn Crohn's disease storyline.

Chapter Eleven

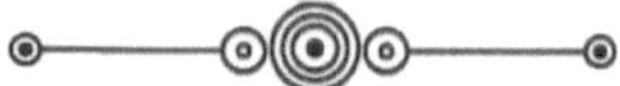

One Tuesday in late August 2007, I was at work at 13 WHAM and I started feeling a strong, sharp pain in the side of my stomach. I was used to feeling some discomfort pretty much all the time, but this felt like something was being jabbed right into my guts. I also still felt my usual sudden urges to have to go to the bathroom, but not much was coming out.

I called Dr. Griswold's office and said that I felt like I was taking a turn for the worse, and I asked if I could get in to see him. I got an appointment for that Thursday, two days away. I really struggled to make it through those next couple of days, but as usual, I did not call in sick to work. Meanwhile, Amanda was getting ready to go out of town. She was going to take a long weekend and go visit her friend Jen back in Virginia. Then she saw how off I was feeling.

"I'm going to call Jen and say I'm not coming," Amanda said. "You're really not doing well."

"No, no, don't do that," I insisted. "I'm fine. If you canceled plans any time I wasn't feeling good, you'd never do anything. I'll see Dr. Griswold and get this straightened out." At my insistence and reassurance, Amanda left for Virginia.

On Thursday, after making it through my usual early-morning shift at 13 WHAM, I went in to see Dr. Griswold. His office was in a large complex of other medical professionals. As I sat in the waiting room, my guts were in knots. I still felt the sharp pain, like I had razor blades trying to make their way through my digestive tract. There was no restroom visible in the small waiting area. I really needed to go sit on the toilet and try to get some relief. I left the waiting room and went out into the hallway, looking for a bathroom. I found one just down the hall from Griswold's office, but to my alarm, it was locked.

I went back to Griswold's waiting room. There was another patient at the window being checked in. I stood awkwardly off to the side until she had been signed in, and then discreetly walked up to the window and asked the office assistant, "Is there a restroom nearby that I can use?"

"Yes, there's one down the hall, but you need a key," she said. She slid open her desk drawer and handed me the key to the bathroom.

I thought, *How cruel and insensitive is it to have a gastroenterologist's office where you need to go down the hall, with a key, to use the bathroom?* They should have had toilets right in the middle of the waiting room as far as I was concerned! I took the key, ran to the bathroom, and spent a couple of minutes trying to get the razor blades to leave my body. I got some out, and there was blood in the bowl.

When I finally got in to see Dr. Griswold, my exam was short. I talked to him about how much pain I was in, and how this was different and much worse than what my usual day-to-day Crohn's symptoms were like. I told him about the blood that had been in my stool just now. He was concerned enough to send me to the emergency room to get checked out. It made me wonder if that's what I should have done two days ago when I called him instead of waiting for an office visit, only for him to tell me to go to the ER.

At the emergency room, they gave me a CT scan, which revealed that the whole left side of my intestines were severely inflamed. They decided to admit me to the hospital overnight and put me on an IV, awaiting further instructions from Dr. Griswold.

When I was admitted to my room, the first thing I did was run to the bathroom and evacuate my bowels again. I still had the sharp pain in my intestines, and even though it was painful, at least sitting on the toilet helped things move. Plus, after being surrounded by technicians and having to lay still on a table to get the CT scan done, it felt good to just be in the bathroom and have some privacy. That is, until there was a knock on the bathroom door.

"Russell?" a low male voice said through the door.

"Yeah?" I replied.

"Did you have a bowel movement?" the voice asked.

"Yes...?" I replied.

"Can I see it?" the voice asked.

What the hell was happening? For some reason, I envisioned some kind of perverted Hunchback of Notre Dame–looking character outside my bathroom door who had a fetish for looking at people's feces. In reality, it was just a nurse who I guess had the pleasure of checking my stool to make sure there wasn't blood in it. He told me that any time I had a bowel movement to please call someone to look at it before I flushed it. This gave me anxiety because my bowel movements tended to be very frequent, and pressing a call button to make a public announcement about it was the last thing I wanted to do.

Once I got a little more settled in, I called Amanda and let her know what was going on. Of course, she felt terrible that she was out of town and now I was in the hospital. There was a mix of guilt over not being there and also maybe a little bit of "I told you so" frustration with me since I had insisted she still go on her trip when she had already felt like she shouldn't.

I set my alarm on my phone to wake me up at 3:30 a.m., so I could call in sick for my shift at 13 WHAM. I did not tell them I was in the hospital, just that I was not feeling well. Because I was part time and had no sick or vacation time, this would be a day I did not get paid for.

The next day, Friday, a doctor on staff stopped in and told me he had spoken to Dr. Griswold about my CT scan and that he was going to put me on prednisone. From everything I had read about treatment for Crohn's disease, I knew that this was a steroid commonly used to treat inflammation. I had read about a bunch of side effects that tended to come along with it, like irritability, increased appetite, weight gain, acne, and something referred to as "moon face." I was looking forward to exactly none of these side effects, but honestly the one that worried me the most was the increased appetite. What a terrible side effect for someone who could barely eat anything! What was I going to do if this drug made me hungry all the time?

Dr. Griswold was starting me off with a dose of 40 mg per day. The doctor on call who I spoke to said I should follow up with Dr. Griswold once I was out of the hospital, and that we could discuss gradually tapering me off of the prednisone. It made me feel a little better to know the plan was already to start getting me off of it as soon as we could. I was also hopeful that this stuff would do the trick and get my inflammation back down in short order. As much as I was hesitant to be on the steroid in the first place, maybe it would at least give me some quick relief from my pain.

In the meantime, they wanted to keep me in the hospital for observation. This would mean calling in sick to Sam's Club on Saturday as well.

Despite the fact that the staff needed to routinely examine my excrement every time I took a crap, there was something comforting about being in the hospital. I spent every minute of every day in public trying desperately to hide my disease, to hide how sick I was always feeling. Now I was in a place where everyone not only knew, but it was literally their job to try to help me get better. It felt safe, like I didn't have to hide my secret. It felt like it was okay to be sick now.

Saturday morning, I called Sam's Club and talked to Coach John. I don't know why, but I told him I was in the hospital rather than just saying I was sick like I had with 13 WHAM. I think it may have partially been because I was at Sam's so rarely anyway, only working on the weekends, as well as being one of only a few people who were trained to work in the accounting office, that calling in sick felt like a big deal. And since I had my health insurance through Sam's, I felt like I really needed a good reason to miss a shift there. I always felt like at any moment they could say, do we really need to keep this guy around for just two days a week?

"Hey, Coach John," I said. "It's Russ Dimino."

"Hey, Russ," he replied hesitantly. I'm sure any manager who took a call from an employee knew they were going to say they weren't coming in to work.

"I'm not going to be able to make it in today. I'm actually in the hospital right now."

"You're in the *hospital*?" He obviously wasn't expecting that. "Is everything okay?"

"Yeah," I said. "I, um. I have Crohn's disease," I explained. "I'm having a pretty bad flare-up of it." Even as I was saying the words, I thought back to that time at the hospital in Virginia when I'd asked for a doctor's note explaining why I was there, and the physician had said I didn't have to tell my employer that. I knew I didn't have to tell Coach John that I had Crohn's disease, but I did anyway.

"Oh man, I'm sorry to hear that," he said, sounding genuinely sympathetic. "Hey, Russ, hold on a second, okay?"

"Okay..."

I could hear him set the phone down, and I heard some papers shuffling around like he was looking for something.

"Hey, Russ, your eval is due today. I have to give it to you," Coach John said when he came back to the phone, referring to my annual performance evaluation.

"Oh…" I said.

"What hospital are you at?" he asked.

"Um. I'm at Rochester General," I said.

"Okay. I'm going to stop by and see you if that's okay," he said.

"Uh. Sure, that's fine…" I said.

At Sam's Club, it was a real serious offense if a manager did not give you your annual evaluation on time. Getting your eval late would mean that your raise, if you got one, would go into effect late, and I imagine that the company wanted to avoid any potential lawsuits or anything like that from employees who felt they had missed out on wages due to getting a late review. Because of that, as legend has it, a manager could actually be fired for giving an employee their eval late. So Coach John came and visited me at Rochester General Hospital and gave me my annual performance review in my hospital room. I was in a hospital gown, looked and felt like shit, had not showered since Thursday, and now had my manager sitting in a chair next to my hospital bed reading me an evaluation of my work. It was bizarre.

The good news was that my review was glowingly positive, I was getting a forty-cent-per-hour raise, and they were even going to pay me for the fifteen minutes that it took for him to give me my eval in the hospital. What a world!

My parents also came and visited me and were with me most of the day on Saturday. I was starting to feel better, and I was hopeful that I was going home that day, and in fact the nurses had said a few times that I probably would. I was looking forward to sleeping in my own bed. I would take the day off from Sam's Club again tomorrow (since my manager had just seen me in the hospital, I was pretty sure me taking another day off would be expected) and just have a quiet day at home all by myself on Sunday. That sounded like heaven.

But some of the readings they were getting on my bloodwork were concerning and indicated my inflammation was still higher than it should be. The doctor on call came in and told me that they wanted to keep me one more day for observation. It was a crushing blow. My hope of one simple day at home by myself was apparently too much to ask.

My parents saw how disappointed I was to get the news that I would not be going home. They made it their mission to raise my spirits. They made a run back to my apartment and came back to the hospital with my laptop and a stack of comic books. It was a game changer to have some entertainment at my disposal while I was confined to the hospital bed. I also took a shower. I had been holding off on taking one just because it's such a pain—they have to unhook you from the monitors and the IV stuff, cover up the IV plug that's in your hand, yadda yadda yadda. But it was worth it. It helped me feel more human again.

I was finally discharged from the hospital on Sunday. I made sure to go to bed early that night.

I went right back to my 3:30 a.m. shift at 13 WHAM on Monday morning.

Chapter Twelve

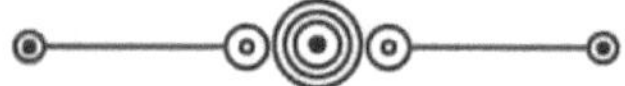

There had been a lot of changes in my life in rapid succession at this point, and I didn't feel like I was in control of many of them. I was working seven days a week and going to bed early most nights, which meant that Amanda and I were not getting much time together.

My health was a roller-coaster ride that I hadn't wanted to get on in the first place. I was on multiple medications, including the newly prescribed prednisone, and still not achieving anything close to what I would consider remission from my Crohn's disease. With so much of my own life feeling like it was slipping through my fingers, I decided to grab one very specific element that was vitally important to me and hold it close, to solidify it so it wouldn't evaporate like water on a summer day. Something I felt that I had been lucky not to lose already.

I was going to ask Amanda to marry me.

In the guise of simply planning a special getaway, I suggested we go up to Niagara Falls for a few days. It was less than a two-hour drive, so an easy destination for a long weekend. I took the days off from Sam's Club, which I was a little reluctant to do after just missing work there a couple of weeks back, but I figured I still had some sympathy built up from those guys since Coach John had literally seen me in a hospital bed.

We drove up to Niagara Falls, Ontario. I surprised Amanda by getting us a gorgeous room at the Embassy Suites hotel with a whirlpool tub and a huge picture window overlooking the falls. The look of awe on Amanda's face when we walked into the room was like a kid coming downstairs on Christmas morning and seeing an enormous pile of presents under the tree. She'd had no idea this was where we were going to be staying.

As part of our hotel stay, we also got shuttle passes to get around Clifton Hill, which is a tourist area near the falls with lots of museums and other fun attractions. Once we were checked into the hotel, we headed out to see the sights. Clifton Hill was a big boardwalk full of bright lights and bustling activity. A colossal Frankenstein's monster holding a huge hamburger overlooked both a haunted house and a Burger King, tying those mismatched destinations together. An arcade with flashing lights and blaring sirens beckoned you to come in and try to win a prize. The Movieland Wax Museum offered the opportunity to pose next to lifelike statues of everyone from Beyoncé to the Terminator. A 4-D simulation ride let you experience wild adventures like being perched precariously on the edge of a perilous cliff. There were dozens of restaurants to choose from, and to satisfy your sweet tooth there was Hershey's Chocolate World, a 7,000-square-foot retail store devoted to candy.

All of this pales in comparison to the sight of the falls themselves. We are a bit spoiled in Upstate New York in that this veritable wonder of the world is just an afternoon's drive away. They really are a spectacle that needs to be seen to be believed. Niagara Falls is actually comprised of three distinct waterfalls: the Horseshoe Falls, the American Falls, and the (comparatively) much smaller Bridal Veil Falls. Every second, more than 750,000 gallons of water gushes over the three falls combined.

On the Canadian side, you can stand across from them and see all of them at once. From the U.S., you don't get to experience the full panoramic view of the three waterfalls, but you can get right up close to the American Falls, if you are so inclined. The majesty of it is overwhelming. The sheer power of Mother Nature is awe-inspiring. Amanda and I stood side by side, holding hands as we looked out at the wonderous sight of the falls as the sun began to set. A misty drizzle overtook the world around us, making it feel like a cool and breezy dreamscape as the sky turned soft shades of purple and orange. Amanda rested her head on my shoulder and gently squeezed my hand. For this moment in time, everything felt peaceful.

You might be wondering how I was managing my Crohn's symptoms through all of this. Being on prednisone had quieted things down in my gut, at least to the extent that the shooting pain was gone and I no longer had blood in my stool. It did not take away the sudden trips to the bathroom that I still was having to make a couple dozen times a day, every day.

To get through the weekend, I had taken some Imodium. This was a trick I could do only so often, and it always came with a price. Taking Imodium slowed things down in my gut so that I did not have to go so often or so urgently, but doing this would "back things up" so that once I stopped taking it, I would ultimately have more urgency and more discomfort when my system fired back up in a day or so. This was not pleasant, but it allowed me to live a normal life for a brief period of time when needed.

I had told Amanda ahead of time to bring one "dress-up" outfit because we were going out to a nice dinner on Saturday night. She wore a low-cut black blouse and a floral-print skirt and looked positively radiant. I wore a black-and-white-striped button-down shirt and khaki pants and looked pretty good, if I say so myself. We had dinner at the Keg Steakhouse, which was a restaurant on the ninth floor of the hotel. Much like the room we were staying in, the restaurant had floor-to-ceiling windows with a spectacular view of the falls. We had a table for two right next to one of the windows. Everything about it felt magical.

I was nervous, though, and Amanda could tell. She kept asking me if I felt okay, chalking my edginess up to my Crohn's. I kept insisting I was fine, all the while checking my pocket over and over for the ring box I had stowed there. I had bought the ring a few weeks earlier; the fact that I only worked until 12:30 p.m. at the latest on weekdays had afforded me the luxury of being able to go ring-shopping during the day while Amanda was at work. My mom and sister had come with me on a few of my shopping excursions for help and advice.

My sister, by the way, was over-the-moon excited that I was going to ask Amanda to marry me. When I was thinking of popping the question, I had asked Val, "So what do you think of Amanda?" She stared at me blankly for a beat, then realized why I was asking. "Oh my God!" she exclaimed. "I freaking love her!" The anticipation of this night had been building, not just for me, but for my emotionally-invested family members as well. But now, as Amanda and I sat in the restaurant and the big night was finally here, I was convinced that the ring box was going to spontaneously disappear from my pocket.

I was also anxious because there was another part of my plan that I was hoping to pull off, and I wasn't sure exactly how to execute it. I had my camera with me, and I was hoping to have someone take a photo of me popping the question. Keep in mind this was 2007, in the days well before everybody having a smartphone at their disposal. I just wanted everything to go perfectly. That, along with the fact that dining out at a restaurant was not really my element at all these days, was definitely making me feel a bit on edge.

After we ordered our food, I ran to the bathroom. Despite the Imodium having slowed things down, I did still have to go. There was a twisting in my guts as I sat down on the bowl. A tense, kind of kneading sensation in my intestines, like trying to wring a few drops of toothpaste out of a stubborn tube. I bent over and put my head in my hands as I let my bowels do what they needed to do. I gritted my teeth.

"Ugh, I don't need this right now," I muttered. Like there was ever a time that I needed it. I shook my head at the situation. Was it not enough to just be anxious about proposing to my girl? Why did I also have to juggle the fact that my stupid Crohn's disease could wreak havoc with my stomach at any moment? Anyone else would be able to just enjoy a delicious steak dinner. I had to worry about every morsel of food that went into my mouth. The injustice of it made me so mad. I would have given anything to just worry about the things that "normal" people worried about.

I finished up in the bathroom and went back to the table, telling myself that everything was going to be fine. I was determined not to let the evening get ruined.

The food was amazing. I hadn't had a steak and baked potato in so long. It felt like a dangerous indulgence. My Crohn's disease demon lurked over my shoulder again, watching me take each succulent bite with a sardonic smile. Did I deserve any of this? Not just the delicious food, but the gorgeous girl and the life I was going to try to build with her? Every time I felt myself getting close to what I wanted, my disease seemed determined to destroy my dreams. I tried to shut out those doubts and just be present with Amanda.

As we were finishing up the meal, Amanda excused herself to go to the restroom. This was my chance. As soon as she was out of sight, I flagged down our waitress. She came over to the table.

"Hey!" I said. "I need to ask you a huge favor. I'm going to propose to my girlfriend here tonight."

"You *are*?" Her eyes lit up and she grinned excitedly. She was so psyched already that you would have thought she was a friend who had known us for years.

"Yes! I have my camera here with me," I said, holding it up. "When she comes back to the table, I'm going to ask you to take a picture of us. Then, after you take the picture, I'm going to get down on one knee with the ring, and I need you to keep taking pictures."

"All right!" she said. "This is so exciting!" She looked like she was about to start jumping up and down. I had probably just made this girl's night. I was glad she was so eager to help—I could tell I had recruited the right person. She assured me she would be back in a few minutes to carry out the plan. She practically skipped away.

Amanda came back to the table, and I tried to act nonchalant. By now it had gotten dark outside. The view outside the surrounding windows was even more stunning, as the falls were lit up with colored lights, casting them in cool blue, purple, and green hues that looked like something straight out of a fairy tale. We admired the view and commented on how great the meal had been. I casually remarked that when the waitress came back we should ask her to take a picture of us. I checked my pocket for the thousandth time.

Our waitress deserved to be nominated for an Oscar for how calm and casual she acted when she returned to the table to ask if we needed anything else. I asked her if she would mind taking a picture of us.

"Sure!" she said. I handed her my camera.

I put my hand on top of Amanda's. We leaned toward each other across the table and smiled. The waitress snapped a picture.

"Amanda," I said, "I need to ask you something."

I got up from the table and knelt down on one knee in front of her. Her jaw dropped. There was a flash as the waitress snapped another pic.

"Over these past few years, we have spent a lot of time together, and we've also spent a lot of time apart," I continued. "I know that I don't ever want us to be apart again." I reached into my pocket. The ring was still there, fortunately. I pulled out the ring box, carefully opened it, and held it aloft. There was the flash of another photo being taken. Amanda's mouth was still agape, but she was also grinning ear to ear. It doesn't seem like you should be able to do both of those things at the same time, but she was. "Amanda Rose, will you marry me?" I asked. *Flash.*

Without a moment's hesitation, her reply was, "Of course I will!"

I took the ring out of the box and slid it onto her finger. *Flash.*

Cheers and applause broke out all around us. I looked around and realized that everyone in the restaurant was looking at us and clapping. I had been so intently focused on this moment that I had almost forgotten there were other people around. Some people even came over to shake my hand, and two women came up to Amanda and told her they cried when I asked her.

The waitress handed me my camera back as another waiter came over with two glasses of champagne and a single long-stem red rose and placed them on the table. "Congratulations!" our waitress said with a huge gin. "Please enjoy some champagne on us!"

Amanda was positively beaming. She kept looking at the ring with a huge smile. She picked up the rose off of the table and smelled it, as if trying to take in every sensory element of the moment. My excitement was overshadowed by an overwhelming feeling of relief.

As a side note, it had been suggested to me multiple times that being nervous about the upcoming proposal was what caused the flare-up that landed me in the hospital prior to this. Stress is certainly a factor when it comes to Crohn's and ulcerative colitis and can contribute to exacerbating symptoms. But I think to say that me being anxious about proposing was what landed me in the hospital is an oversimplification at best.

With the old expression "the straw that broke the camel's back," it's not the single straw that busts the camel's hump, it's the accumulation of everything the beast is carrying. I cannot emphasize to you enough that I was stretching myself far too thin, working two jobs and not getting enough sleep. I worried about not having access to a bathroom when I needed it. I worried about every bite of food that went into my mouth. I worried about how much I was worrying.

If you asked me at the time if I was worried about proposing to Amanda, I would have quite honestly said no. I was excited to do it, and I was very confident that she would say yes. It was something I was looking forward to doing. There was certainly some underlying anxiety, as you have just read, about getting the moment just right. But compared to the anxiety I felt about pretty much everything all the time, it was negligible, or at least it felt different. Did having one more thing to worry about push me over the edge and put me in the hospital? I don't know.

That is one of the most frustrating things about Crohn's, though. When your symptoms take a turn for the worse, people around you tend to ask, "What do you think caused this? What did you do differently? What did you eat?" And surely they mean well in asking that. They want to help you pinpoint what is making your symptoms worse so you can avoid it in the future and stay well.

But it is almost never that simple. If it was, no one would be sick.

Chapter Thirteen

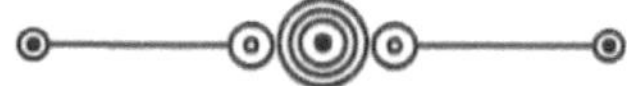

In mid-September 2007, my mom and dad, my brother, my sister, and Amanda and I took part in the Guts and Glory walk, a walk-a-thon fundraiser for the Crohn's and Colitis Foundation of America. Our team name was the Crohn's Busters. We raised money mostly through soliciting online donations, and the six of us together raised $1,700. The money raised went toward medical research, as well as programs to improve the quality of life for people suffering from Crohn's and ulcerative colitis. I remember reading that one of the programs included was a summer camp for children. As hard as it was for me being an adult with Crohn's, I could not imagine trying to cope with it as a kid.

The walk took place on the campus of Monroe Community College. There were balloons and cones marking off the trail for the walk. There were lots of vendors where you could get things to eat, like hotdogs or popcorn. This struck me as a bit strange, seeing as popcorn was one of the number one foods you should not eat if you have Crohn's because it is so hard to digest. Sure, not every person here actually had the disease, but it seemed odd and a little insensitive. Like serving cake and ice cream at a diabetes walk.

What struck me the most, though, was the sheer number of people there. I don't know what I expected, but the fact that there were hundreds of people in attendance really opened my eyes to the fact that this disease impacted more people than I thought. Before my diagnosis, I had never even heard of Crohn's disease. Why weren't more people talking about it?

Of course, I knew why. It was the same reason no one I worked with knew I had Crohn's. The symptoms were so embarrassing. Who wanted to admit they had a disease that gave them urgent, painful, unpredictable poops? But being surrounded by other people who had the disease, along with family members who loved and supported them, along with my own family who loved and supported me, made me feel less alone. The fact that we were all there to raise money for this cause gave me hope.

I thought back to what Dr. Griswold had said about the possibility of a cure in my lifetime. Could that possibly come true? (And could they hurry it up a little?)

Dr. Griswold wanted to try to taper me off of prednisone. I had started in the hospital at 40 mg per day. They came in 5 mg pills, so I took four in the morning and four in the evening. After about a week, Dr. Griswold had me taper it down so I was taking 35 mg per day: four pills in the morning and three in the evening. Another week after that, I went down to 30 mg per day, which was three pills in the morning and three in the evening. The next week, 25 mg. The next week, 20 mg. This was in addition to the Pentasa that I was still taking.

By mid-October, I was down to a dose of 12.5 mg per day, which was one and a half pills in the morning—I had to buy a pill splitter to cut one of them in half—and one in the evening. Around this time, I noticed blood showing up in my stool again and more discomfort whenever I was going to the bathroom. I continued tapering the prednisone anyway.

By the end of October, I was down to one pill in the morning and half a pill in the evening (7.5 mg), and things were becoming unbearable. I was having urgent, liquidy, painful bowel movements that often had blood in them. I called Dr. Griswold's office. Rather than even telling me to come in, he told me to up the prednisone back to 30 mg.

I definitely noticed a difference when I was on the higher dose of prednisone. While it didn't completely take my symptoms away, it at least made them manageable. The sharp pain and discomfort would go away. I would still have moments where I needed to get to a bathroom quickly, but I wasn't in agony, and it didn't feel like I was trying to pass a grenade that was in the process of exploding. It took a toll on my mood at higher doses, though. I felt irritable, like I was always on edge. I'd snap at Amanda for no reason. It was ironic that I felt physically better and yet mentally I became Oscar the Grouch.

Dr. Griswold said we would need to taper the prednisone much more gradually than we had tried to initially. I stayed at 30 mg for two weeks, then dropped it by only half a pill to 27.5 mg. I would continue to taper off by half a pill every two weeks.

This time I only made it down to 20 mg. By the middle of December, the blood and the painful urgency were back. I called Dr. Griswold, and he bumped me back up to 30 mg again.

I was in a rough place. I'd been hopeful that I'd get on and off the prednisone quickly, but that didn't seem like it was going to be the case. Obviously what we were doing was not working. I was desperate to find something that would improve my quality of life and feeling depressed about my current state.

My mother, God bless her, never stopped researching ways to help me get my disease under control. She was on every website, reading every article, checking every book out of the library that might offer the secret to alleviating my pain. She came across one book in particular that touted a grain-free diet that was known to help people with Crohn's, colitis, celiac disease, diverticulitis, and even cystic fibrosis reduce or eliminate their symptoms and lead normal lives. This book had a strong following on the web, and there was a message board where people could reach out for support and guidance from others who had tried the diet or were going through it along with them.

As I stated previously, I am not going to say what the book was or give a lot of details about the diet here. I don't want to give the impression that because something did not work for me, it's not legit. Based on what I saw on the forums, this diet did seem to be genuinely helpful to a lot of people. If you are inclined to seek it out, you can probably figure it out based on what I am describing and a little research of your own.

With this diet, you cut out all grains, all dairy, anything canned or processed, and all sugar. That right there is going to be a shock to anyone's system if you have never cut those foods out before. Instead, you are eating unprocessed meat, fish, eggs, nuts, and there was a recipe for a homemade yogurt that was integral to the diet, as the yogurt was a part of several other recommended recipes in the back of the book.

My mom got me a copy of the book. I was willing to give it a try. It started out much like the diet I had tried back in Virginia, by having you eliminate everything from your diet except a few very specific things. For the first five days or so, you ate nothing but homemade chicken broth, cooked (soft) carrots, and broiled meat. In a way, I really was fine with this. A few days of not thinking or stressing about what to eat and keeping it simple was its own freedom in a way.

Then I promptly messed everything up by skipping too far into the diet too quickly.

You will note that I said that nuts were okay to eat on this diet. What I failed to understand was that nuts only came into play much later on, after your guts have healed quite a bit and are able to handle them. Nuts are high in fiber and can be difficult to digest. They offer a lot of protein and unsaturated fats, but they are not easy for your digestive system to process if it's already in rough shape. I was so eager to dive into the diet that I did not read the book with the intent to really understand this. I went to the back of the book to find recipes that I assumed would make me better. The first thing I made was a batch of muffins that involved chopping up almonds in a food processor to make my own almond flour.

I was in agony after I ate them. My intestines were being scraped raw with sandpaper. I was digesting thumbtacks. It was excruciating, and I didn't know how to make it stop. I ended up having to call in sick to 13 WHAM, which was something I almost never did, no matter how bad I was feeling.

Upon more careful reading of the book, I now understood that I had been an idiot, and any of the recipes with nuts were for *after* your gut was healed and healthy. I had just set myself back significantly in the process. Back to broth for me.

My diet quickly became the homemade broth with chicken and soft carrots, and plain scrambled eggs. The almond incident had been such a scare that I was afraid to progress to the next stage of the diet. Even after reading the book much more carefully, I was so gun-shy that I didn't want to step off the starting line. I would make a big batch of the chicken soup about once a week and then just warm it up a bowl at a time throughout the week. It was soothing, comforting, and most of all, it was safe. I would usually make scrambled eggs when I got home from work at the station and eat soup at dinnertime. Those two meager meals were about all I felt comfortable eating for a long time.

At the gentle encouragement of Amanda, I did finally branch out and try to add a couple of other simple things to the diet: broiled plain hamburgers—no bun, no condiments, no seasoning, just broiled ground beef—and broiled tilapia. Amanda can't stand the smell of any kind of seafood, but to her credit, she never complained when I would make tilapia. I tried to do it sparingly and when she was not around, and to be fair, tilapia doesn't tend to have as strong of a fishy smell as other kinds of seafood might.

Still, I knew she didn't like it, but she never complained. I'm sure she could not bring herself to say anything unkind about the food I was actually willing to eat when my diet was so limited.

It's really amazing how often food is offered to you when you are trying to avoid it. Someone in the business office at Sam's Club would sometimes bring in donuts or cookie cake for everyone. I'd usually say that I had just eaten and that maybe I'd grab some later if there was any left.

At 13 WHAM, every week on the CW morning show we had a segment called Soul Plates, where Jerry Manley from the Flour City Diner and Miss Betty of Miss Betty's Slammin' Sauces would come in and make a savory Southern-style dish live on the air. It was the crew's favorite day of the week, because after the segment was over, there would always be plenty for everyone to dig into and enjoy.

Everyone except me. But I didn't want everyone to know my secret. I didn't want people to know I was sick and feel bad for me. So when it was time to eat, I would either just disappear very quickly or sometimes even take some food and pretend to eat it until I could discreetly dispose of it. I never took very much when I did that, and I only did it when there was way more than enough to go around. I hated that I was being wasteful and throwing out food that was undoubtedly absolutely delicious. It always smelled amazing, and everyone would be raving about how good the food was.

People would be coming into the studio from sub-control or the pit to grab a plate during the commercial break. I knew if I said, "I can't have any because I have Crohn's disease and I'm on a special diet," I would receive looks of pity and probably have a lot of questions to answer, and I just didn't want that. I wanted to fade into the background. I honestly didn't even feel bad that I couldn't eat the food. I just wanted to disappear.

Ironically, I was not the only employee at 13 WHAM who had Crohn's. One of the photographers—I will call him Nate—also had it, and everyone knew. He seemed to have it pretty well under control, from what I could tell. You would think this would have been an amazing connection for me to have. Someone who worked at the same place that I did, who had the same disease that I had, and who seemed to have figured out how to manage his symptoms. I should talk to him and ask how he did it, right?

Nope. I was too timid to do it. Nate was not a guy I crossed paths with a lot. I was on the early-morning shift in the studio; he tended to work more of a nine-to-five and was often out on assignment shooting video footage. I did see him sometimes when he would be in the newsroom or in an edit bay working on something. Looking back now, it's easy for me to say I should have gone up to him and introduced myself. He seemed like a very nice guy, and it actually probably would have meant a lot to him to be able to impart any advice that he may have had about managing his disease. Who knows, maybe he could have used someone to commiserate with too. Just because it seemed to me like he was doing well didn't mean he really was. Maybe he had just gotten good at hiding his pain, just like me.

But at that time, when it was still such a taboo thing for me and I was so intent on keeping it a secret, striking up a conversation about it with a relative stranger seemed impossible.

One day on the morning show, we actually had an in-studio interview with a doctor who talked about Crohn's disease. During the course of the interview, Evan mentioned that we had someone on staff with Crohn's.

When I got home from work that day, my mom called me. "I heard Evan mention that there was someone on staff with Crohn's! I didn't know you finally told everyone!"

"Oh, he wasn't talking about me," I said. "There is another guy who works at the station, Nate, who has Crohn's too."

"Well, why is it okay for everyone to know that Nate has Crohn's, but you don't want them to know that you have it?"

"I don't know, Mom. I just don't."

I actually did hear a couple of the other photographers talking about Nate one time when he was not around, and that was actually how I first learned that he had Crohn's. They were not even saying anything bad. I think one of them said something like, "Did you know Nate has Crohn's disease? All the guy can eat is boiled chicken." It was said in sort of a pitying, how-awful-that-must-be kind of way. And I just didn't want anyone to talk about me like that or think of me that way.

Would it have been any worse than how things currently were, though? Being quiet, staying in the background, not making friends with anyone, and pretending to eat things was not exactly a great time. I think I just let myself keep thinking that I was going to get healthy any day now. That this way of life was only temporary. That soon things would be different and I would be able to eat normally and hang out with everyone. Why tell them I was sick if I wasn't going to be sick much longer?

I continued to make the chicken soup every week. One evening, I had just finished making a huge batch of it, and I sat down with Amanda to eat dinner. I took one sip of the soup, and something did not taste right. It tasted sweet and kind of… tangy? It didn't make sense. I knew exactly what the soup was supposed to taste like, and this wasn't it. I took another slurp of it. What the heck did it taste like?

You know how sometimes you do things on autopilot that don't register at all at the time, but then your brain replays it later on and reminds you of what you did? I had a flashback to when I had been putting the garlic powder into the broth. My unconscious mind was able to cue it up like a CSI playing back footage of a crime scene. I hadn't grabbed the garlic powder. The little CSI guy in my brain zoomed in and enhanced the label on the seasoning container. I had put cinnamon into the broth instead.

It tasted terrible. The soup was supposed to be salty, not sweet. I couldn't eat it.

Amanda asked what was wrong and why I was not eating. I was too embarrassed to tell her that I had ruined a huge pot of soup with a dumb mistake. Instead I just said I wasn't very hungry. I literally had not eaten anything all day and had spent a couple of hours on a batch of soup that was supposed to last me a week.

The diet was a real pain to keep up with, and to be honest, I was not seeing a ton of improvement from it. In fact, I was getting true diarrhea more often than I usually did, lots of loose, watery stools. I took to the internet and asked on one of the message boards devoted to this diet if that was normal.

"You are experiencing what is called 'die off,'" one of the moderators responded to my post. "That's good, it means you are making progress. The bad bacteria in your gut are dying off, and it is common to have those kinds of symptoms while that is happening."

This was not great news to me.

"So, am I understanding correctly that it's normal to feel worse before I feel better?" I asked.

"Yes, absolutely," the moderator replied.

I didn't know if I could handle feeling worse before I felt better. Couldn't anything make me feel *better* before I felt better?

I continued sticking with the diet, really hoping that a turning point was just around the corner. My mom bought a special yogurt maker that was used to make the yogurt recipe that was integral to some of the other recipes in the book, as well as promoting healthy bacteria to grow in your gut even when eaten on its own. She would give me some yogurt to take home every time I saw her.

There was a cheesecake recipe you could make with the yogurt, vanilla extract, honey, eggs, and lemon juice; I made it a few times. It did not taste quite like "real" cheesecake, but it was pretty good, and it felt incredible to eat something resembling a dessert. Other than that, though, I did not deviate much from soup, eggs, broiled burgers, and broiled tilapia. In theory, I should have been advancing through the diet, but I still just could not bring myself to do much more.

After sticking with this for a few months, I decided to try another recipe in the book. I tried to make a grape juice gelatin, which was kind of like an all-natural grape Jell-O that you make from scratch. The book specifically indicated that it was intended for the introductory phase of the diet, so I figured it could not be that risky to try.

I took one bite of the gelatin, and I was immediately in the bathroom with explosive diarrhea.

Now, I am a pretty logical person. (Although I'm sure some portions of this book point pretty strongly to the contrary.) I know that when you take one bite of something, it does not instantly travel through your whole digestive tract and give you diarrhea within moments of eating it.

But I also have experienced firsthand that sometimes you can introduce something into your system and it's like throwing a rock into a pond—there are ripples that spread out and make little waves in the water, radiating out from where the rock actually hit. I truly believe that a sensitive digestive system can act very much the same way, especially one that already has a hairpin trigger due to being inflamed. I think you can eat something that has not even hit your stomach yet that makes your whole system say "NOPE" and it starts smashing every eject button it can reach.

This is what happened to me with the gelatin. I cannot tell you if I did something wrong with how I made it, or if there was a strong mental component that was just insanely nervous about me trying something new and it threw my bowels into a red alert as the gelatin was still coming in for a landing. All I knew was I was on the bowl with my legs shaking and a brown Mount Vesuvius erupting from my sphincter after putting only one bite of grape gelatin down the hatch.

I could not do this. I couldn't stay with this diet. I had to find something else.

I was afraid to tell my mom that I was stopping the diet. I felt like I would be letting her down somehow. She had been the one to find this book and all the information about the diet, and she made the yogurt for me and everything. I was worried about disappointing her, or that maybe she would think I hadn't given it enough of a chance and she would try to talk me into keeping it going.

Of course, that was not how she reacted at all, and I should have known better. She felt bad that the diet hadn't helped me and did not want me to keep doing something that wasn't working out. She jumped right back into research mode and began looking for another diet to try instead.

We have to—and we will!—get you back to where eating is a joyful, pleasurable experience! she wrote to me in an email. *That, in itself, is part of the healing process!*

This made me realize how much my attitude toward food had changed. The idea of eating for enjoyment or pleasure seemed foreign to me now. I thought about how often food was involved in social norms and associated with things that were supposed to be festive or fun. Having a big dinner as a family on Thanksgiving or Christmas. Going on a date to a fancy restaurant. A team-building lunch at work. Going out for ice cream as a reward for a good report card. Hors d'oeuvres at a party. Popcorn at the movies. Cake on your birthday. Even just getting takeout from a favorite diner and bringing it home to eat on the couch while you watch TV. These are all common associations between food and fun.

To me, food was something that was dangerous but necessary. Food was something I had to consider carefully at all times. Something I required but was likely to do me harm. Something I was leery of. Something to fear.

The idea of eating for pleasure was something that other people were so lucky to have, and that they all took for granted. I was honestly not sure I would ever have that again.

For me, the bar was set at wishing I could eat without running to the bathroom or being in pain afterward. My dream was to not have to think so carefully about each and every bite or sip of anything I ate or drank. I was not even aiming for the return of the joy of eating. I just wanted to be rid of the fear of it.

I would have so happily settled for food being something neutral in my life.

Chapter Fourteen

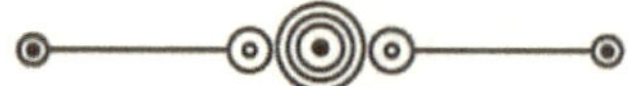

In January 2008, my dad came with me to an appointment with Dr. Griswold. I really felt like Dr. Griswold was not doing enough to help get me on the right track. I couldn't just keep doing the prednisone yo-yo, trying to taper off of it but having to up it again when my inflammation came back. It was time to start exploring some other options, and my dad wanted to come with me to help advocate for that.

Dr. Griswold, for the benefit of my dad, once again opened with the "some asshole has my pen" joke and the explanation of the history of Crohn's disease.

He then talked about the fact that there are generally two different approaches to treating Crohn's disease. Some doctors will throw the strongest possible medications at the patient and then try to slowly back them off and see how far they can back off. That was not the approach he followed, because stronger medications also tended to come with stronger side effects.

The philosophy that he aligned with was to start small and build up to the point that the patient achieves remission. Sometimes you luck out and the patient finds relief with a mild drug. Other times, you need to try something stronger or add layers to the treatment. It was time to add another layer to mine, because he definitely agreed we were not seeing the results that we would want to see. Dr. Griswold talked about three possibilities for treatment: 6-MP, Remicade, and Humira.

Disclaimer: The following descriptions of these medications are based on my own understanding of how they were explained to me. Do not take this as medical advice.

6-MP, aka mercaptopurine, he explained, is a drug that's used to treat autoimmune diseases, including Crohn's, and often used to treat leukemia. It's generally tolerated well by most patients and doesn't often have side effects. The drawback to that medication is that it takes quite a while to build up in the patient's system before it starts to have any benefits, usually about three to six months. I was not in a state where I could wait half a year to get some relief.

Remicade is a TNF-blocker that is also often used to treat Crohn's disease and other autoimmune diseases, including rheumatoid arthritis. Remicade is administered by infusion; you go to the hospital and they give it to you via an IV. The infusions take about two hours. Dr. Griswold explained that Remicade is chimeric, derived from both human and mouse DNA.

Humira is also a TNF-blocker and very effective for treating autoimmune diseases like Crohn's disease. Unlike Remicade, you could administer it yourself at home, via injection, instead of needing to go to the hospital for an infusion. It was "human-human" as opposed to "mouse-human." I don't know the full implications of that, and I'm sure in the medical community this is no big deal, but man, the comparison between injecting myself with something "human-human" vs. having something "mouse-human" slowly dripped into my veins at the hospital seemed like a choice between something unpleasant and something downright horrifying.

Again, *do not* take medical advice from me. If your doctor recommends Remicade or if you're already taking it, I'm so sorry if I'm scaring you. I am just telling you my thoughts and reactions at the time.

Dr. Griswold did caution me that all of these medications can increase your risk of an infection and make it harder for your body to fight one off. Having said all of that, he recommended that we try Humira. Before starting Humira, I would need to be tested for tuberculosis. Dr. Griswold told me to reach out to my primary care physician to schedule a PPD test. He also cautioned me to treat any infections very seriously in the future, and not to hesitate to contact him or my primary doctor in the event of an infection. He wrote me a prescription for Humira and told me that I would come back to his office in a couple of weeks and he would show me how to administer it to myself.

On the drive home, my dad and I talked about the appointment and how we felt it went. We were both glad to hear Dr. Griswold acknowledge that we had not made the progress we were hoping to see so far, and that it was time to take the next step in my treatment. My dad asked if I was comfortable trying a new medication. I said that at this point I knew that I needed something else, and that of the three options Dr. Griswold had discussed with us, Humira seemed to be the best choice.

I dropped the prescription off at a CVS near the apartment. I was still getting my Pentasa filled at Sam's Club for now because it was easy to just keep refilling it, but I cringed at how awkward it was every time I carried out that huge brown to-go bag that looked like I was getting Chinese takeout for a family of four. Getting the Humira filled there too was too much for me to handle. It somehow seemed more reasonable to be getting my meds filled at two different places.

The next day, I got a phone call from CVS.

"Hello, Mr. Dimino?"

"Yes?"

"This is Ryan, the pharmacist from the CVS in Chili. You dropped off a prescription here for Humira?"

"Yes, that's right," I said. I figured they were just calling to tell me it was ready.

"We just wanted to let you know that the total for that prescription comes to $1,100."

There was a long, uncomfortable silence.

"I'm sorry, it comes to how much?"

"$1,100."

"Do you guys need my insurance information?"

"We do have insurance information on file for you in the system, sir," Ryan replied. I'd gotten a few prescriptions filled by CVS before. "Are you still on the Blue Cross Blue Shield?"

"Yes…"

"The $1,100 is after your insurance. Before insurance, it's actually $6,700."

I was stunned. I thought the sticker shock when I had started Pentasa was bad. It was going to cost me a grand to fill this medication—one time.

"Okay," I said slowly. "Thank you for letting me know. Um, don't fill the prescription yet, please. Let me think about what I want to do."

"Okay," the pharmacist said. "Just let us know."

I hung up the phone in disbelief. I had gone from being optimistic at the idea of trying out a new medicine and finally getting some relief to slamming into a brick wall. Could this even possibly be right? Could this medicine really be a thousand bucks *with* insurance?

I called the phone number on the back of my insurance card, explained that my doctor was prescribing Humira, and asked if it was correct that it was really a thousand dollars to fill it once. They double-checked everything and replied politely that, yes, that was the correct amount for that drug with my current coverage.

Just to do my due diligence, and because I was in such complete disbelief that this could be true, I even called around to several area pharmacies to get quotes on how much Humira costs before insurance. CVS had said $6,700. Walmart said $6,722. Walgreens said $6,591. Sam's Club was the lowest at a mere $6,557.

The next person I called was my dad.

"Hey," I said. "I got a call from the pharmacy about that Humira prescription."

"Oh yeah, were they able to get it filled for you?" my dad asked.

"Um. They said it's going to be $1,100. For one refill. *With* my insurance."

"You gotta be kidding me," my dad said in a state of disbelief. "That's *with* insurance?"

"Yeah. Without insurance it's closer to $7,000."

"Un-freaking-believable," my dad said.

"I even called the insurance company to make sure that was right, and they said it is."

"What if you call the doctor's office?" my dad said. "Tell him how much they're saying it's going to be. Maybe they can do something to help you out. I don't know. If he's telling you that's the medicine you should be on, there's gotta be something they can do for you."

"Okay," I said. "Yeah, I can give them a call." All I could think about was when I told Dr. Harvey that my Pentasa was $200. He'd gotten annoyed and said that insurance companies don't care if you lived or died.

"Russ, listen," my dad said. "If that really ends up being how much it costs, I don't want you to worry about it. We will find a way to come up with the money. Mom and I can help you out, we can talk to Grandma, we can talk to Mema and Pepa. We will come up with the money. If this is what it takes to get you feeling better, we will make it happen."

As much as I truly appreciated those words, I knew that I could never do that. I could not ask my family members to go into debt like that for me. I would need to get this medicine filled every *month*. I'd be asking my parents and grandparents to come up with $13,200 a year, every year? I could not put that burden on them. My health was not worth doing that to them. *I* was not worth it. I would just keep suffering in silence rather than drag my family into financial hardship. Plus, what if this medicine didn't even work?

I called Dr. Griswold's office the next morning after work. I spoke to the receptionist and told her that the Humira was going to cost me $1,100.

"Oh my God," she gasped. "Really?" Her surprise surprised me. I guess I assumed this was par for the course for this medicine. The fact that she seemed just as shocked about the cost as I was made me feel like I wasn't crazy.

She said that she would talk to Dr. Griswold about it and then she would get back to me.

Later that day, she called me back.

"Hi, Russ," she said. "I talked to Dr. Griswold, and he said you may be able to get financial assistance for the medication through the pharmaceutical company itself. Try reaching out to the company and ask if there are any programs you can take advantage of to help afford the medication."

I was skeptical. Dr. Harvey's words kept ringing in my ears, and I couldn't help thinking about how naïve I had been when I wrote that letter to my insurance company that had gone unanswered, asking about additional coverage for Pentasa.

I gave my parents the update of what Dr. Griswold's office had recommended. Like I said earlier, one of the great things about my mom is she will research absolutely anything you need information on, usually without even being asked. In this case, my mom was able to find out about a program called MyHumira, where people with no or limited insurance could receive help with the cost of the medication. It was through Abbott, the drug manufacturing company.

I called the phone number for the MyHumira program. I explained my situation, that I had Crohn's disease, that my doctor had prescribed Humira, what kind of insurance I had, and how much it was going to cost me even with my insurance. The woman that I spoke with took some information from me and then put me on hold.

She came back on a few moments later.

"Mr. Dimino?" she said.

"Yes?"

"I'm pleased to inform you that you do qualify for assistance with the MyHumira program," she said. "The first time you fill the prescription, it will cost you $100. For the next six months, we cover the cost of your Humira medication completely; you will not pay anything out of pocket. And then, for the next six months after that, you will pay just $50 per month."

I almost dropped the phone. As much as I was certain I had misunderstood the pharmacist when he first told me it was going to be a thousand bucks, I was even more certain I had to be misunderstanding this woman telling me my medication after the first month would be absolutely free for six months. Finally, I was getting some good news.

The woman went on to say that the MyHumira program could put me in touch with nursing support if I needed assistance with the injection. A nurse could talk me through it over the phone, or potentially even come over to my house to help if I needed it. I thanked this woman over and over again like she had just saved my life. Maybe she had.

I went ahead and got the prescription filled at CVS. With the MyHumira program, it was indeed only $100 for the first month's supply. I carried it out of CVS like I was carrying bars of gold.

In late January, I had another appointment at Dr. Griswold's office, where he showed me how to inject myself with the Humira. Amanda came with me for moral support and so she could also see and understand how it worked. Humira came in a type of injector called a pen, which was a good name for it because it looked like a big fat marker or highlighter.

The first dosage was not one, not two, not three, but *four* injections. Dr. Griswold had me lift up my shirt, and he rubbed a spot on the right side of my abdomen with an alcohol swab. He pressed the pen up against my skin and pushed a button on the bottom of it. There was a click, and I felt the needle plunge into my belly. It stung. I could feel a kind of cold sensation of the medicine coming out of the needle. It wasn't horrible but it wasn't pleasant. After about ten seconds, he was done and asked if I was okay. I said yes, and that it wasn't that bad.

Dr. Griswold did a second injection, this time on the left side of my abdomen.

He let me do the next two. He told me that the abdomen was a good place to do it, but if I didn't like that or if I wanted to use a different spot because my abdomen got too sore, doing it in the middle of the top of my thigh was also a good place. I don't know why, but something about doing it in my thigh actually seemed worse to me.

I pinched a different spot on my abdomen than the two places he had done, back on the right side again but a little higher up. I pinched the skin together between my fingers; the spot just below it where he'd done the first injection was still sore, and even more so as it was pulled tight. I pressed the third pen up against my skin and pushed the button.

There's something so weird about doing it to yourself. There's an instinct that you need to overcome because you know you are the one causing yourself pain. Again, though, it was not unbearable. It was a stinging sensation, but it was tolerable. The feeling of the medicine going into my skin was definitely strange.

I did the fourth injection on the left side of my abdomen, again a little higher than the one Dr. Griswold had done.

By the time we left, my abdomen was pretty tender, but I was feeling hopeful. I wondered how long it would take to start feeling the effects of the Humira. Surely if this medication was so expensive, it had to be powerful stuff. The fact that I'd been able to get it at such an affordable price was a big win. Now I just had to wait for it to work its magic. I was truly optimistic for the first time in a while.

Chapter Fifteen

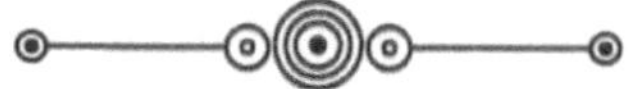

One Saturday evening, Amanda and I and our good friends Tom and Pam went to the movies to see *Sweeney Todd*, starring Johnny Depp and Helena Bonham Carter. We didn't really know anything about it. I think the girls wanted to see it mainly because of Johnny Depp, but Amanda has always been a fan of musicals, so this was something she was really intrigued by. Going out to do anything social was becoming more and more of a rarity for me, because of both my health and my constant work schedule, but a night out with friends sounded nice.

Going out to the movies has always been something I love to do. Escaping into the world of a good film, or even a bad one sometimes, is something magical, and it's what first started simmering that ambition to want to become a filmmaker myself someday. I have a corkboard full of movie ticket stubs from every movie I've gone to see since 1996. Which is why I can tell you that we went to see *Sweeney Todd* on Saturday, January 19, 2008 at 7:05 p.m. at the Henrietta Regal 18, that it was showing in theater 14, and that the tickets cost $9.25 each.

The smell of popcorn was a kind of torture that I had learned to block out. That buttery aroma that seduces your nostrils the moment you walk into the movie theater was a temptation I knew I could not give into. Popcorn is hard to digest and can make inflammation a lot worse. I wondered if I'd ever be able to eat it again in my life. That was hard to think about and made me sad. I couldn't let myself look at it that way. I just told myself I was not going to have it today, rather than thinking about never having it again.

The movie, if you've never seen it or the musical that it's based on, is… well, it is weird. Johnny Depp plays the title character, a barber who slits people's throats with his razor so that his lady friend and partner in crime, Mrs. Lovett (Helena Bonham Carter), can bake them into meat pies. I know that sounds horrific, but it isn't done in a gory or graphic way. It's mostly just bizarre. It's directed by Tim Burton, so that should put it into perspective.

As the movie was building to the crucial moment where Sweeney Todd realizes that Mrs. Lovett has misled him into killing his own wife who he had previously believed to be dead, I felt a familiar sense of discomfort in my guts. I knew that the movie had to be almost over. I tried to tell myself that I could hold it. I'd made it this far! I couldn't get up and go to the bathroom now!

But I did. I had to. I knew I couldn't hold it, not even for a few more minutes. I got up, walked out of the theater stiff-legged, trying to hold everything in, then sprinted down the hall as fast as I could to the nearest restroom. I ran into a stall and barely got my pants down in time before it all came bursting out. It was a painful one, and it was bloody. It was like Sweeney Todd had taken a swipe at my colon with his razor.

As I walked back, I saw a whole bunch of people coming out of one of the theaters. A movie had just gotten out. Then I saw that three of the people coming out of the theater were Tom, Pam, and Amanda. I hadn't realized until just that moment that the theater everyone was filing out of was the one I was on my way back to. Theater 14. I had missed the end of the movie.

To their credit, no one made a big deal about it. In fact, Pam, Tom, and Amanda did not even acknowledge or refer to the fact that I'd had to run out and missed the ending. We just didn't talk about it. Pam and Tom were two of the few friends who knew I had Crohn's disease and who had any idea what I was going through. I had known them both since high school, and Pam and Amanda had been roommates in college. They never judged me. I don't know why I was so afraid that other people would if they knew, but I was.

To this day, I've never seen the ending of *Sweeney Todd*.

At the urging of my parents, I started exploring some more "outside the box" treatment possibilities, including going to an acupuncturist. My grandma's friend had gone to an acupuncturist named Abby in Greece, New York, for a problem she was having with her foot, and she recommended her highly. I figured it was worth a shot. I gave her office a call and spoke with the receptionist there. I said that I was possibly interested in acupuncture, and I was curious if they had experience treating patients with Crohn's disease. I was told to wait for a call back.

Abby returned my call that afternoon. She said that while she did not have experience treating Crohn's specifically, she had treated patients with gastrointestinal issues before, and that she would read up on Crohn's disease and would be glad to treat me if I wanted to come in. The fact that she came recommended from my grandma's friend and that she'd treated gastro issues was promising enough for me. What did I have to lose?

I made an appointment to see Abby. I had a brief moment of worrying about how I would know if it was the Humira or the acupuncture that was helping if I started feeling better. Then I realized I didn't really care. If I could finally start feeling some relief, not knowing which thing got me there would be a problem I could live with.

I went in for my first appointment. The waiting room was quiet and tranquil, with dim lighting and soft music playing. It put me at ease as soon as I walked in. After a few minutes, Abby came out and greeted me and introduced herself. She was short with shoulder-length brown hair. She seemed very nice, and she had a pleasantly calm demeanor.

We went into her office for a few minutes so we could talk about my symptoms and what medications I was taking, and so she could explain a bit about what to expect. Essentially what acupuncture does is open up and stimulate key points in your nervous system that promote the balance of energy and trigger the body's self-healing abilities. She asked if I would be okay with her putting some needles in my abdomen, which can promote digestive healing. I thought about the fact that I was sticking needles into my abdomen already on a regular basis with the

Humira. I told her that I was okay with anything she felt would help me.

Then she took me into the treatment room. It was a small, warm room with a table covered by a couple of white sheets. Again, the lighting was dim and the room was very comfortable. She told me to undress down to my underwear and lay down on the table under the top sheet. She left the room.

When she came back, Abby pulled the sheet up a bit to uncover my legs and down enough to expose my chest and abdomen. She then started very carefully and very deliberately placing the small acupuncture needles into my arms and legs. If you have never had acupuncture done, you may wonder if it hurts. Most of the needles do not. They feel like a slight prick at most, and honestly a lot of them just feel like a little tap. There were a couple that she put in my hand that stung a bit. She put one in the top of my head, and that was the only one that I would say actually did hurt. None of them stung nearly as much as injecting Humira into my belly. The acupuncture needles that she put in my abdomen didn't hurt much at all.

Once the needles had all been properly placed, Abby quietly let me know that she was going to leave for about fifteen minutes. Then she would come back in to "tap" each of the needles, which sort of reactivates them.

She left the room. I closed my eyes and just listened to the soft music. I tried not to think about what I would do if I had to go to the bathroom, which was always in the back of my mind. I would have to either run out of the room in my underwear with needles sticking out of me like a deranged porcupine or shit myself on the acupuncture table. I wasn't sure which option sounded more appealing. I just tried to push it from my mind and relax. In a way, it was nice to have nothing to do but lie there. I tried to focus on my breathing and just let the process do whatever it was going to do.

As promised, she popped back into the room about fifteen or twenty minutes later, quietly asked how I was doing, and then gave each of the needles a gentle tap. Then she left the room again.

After the session was over, Abby came back in and carefully removed each needle one at a time. She asked how I felt. I thought about it for a moment, then answered that I felt relaxed. And it was true. It was certainly a unique experience, and I wasn't sure I completely trusted it just yet, but just some quiet time for some healing and self-care had put me in a calmer state than I was normally in. She said she wanted to see me again the following week.

The next week, 13 WHAM had put me on the evening schedule for a week so that I could get in some director training with the director of the six p.m. and eleven p.m. newscasts. This meant my hours were completely flipped—instead of working 3:30 a.m. to 12:30 p.m., I'd be working three p.m. until midnight. Now I would have to make some adjustments to my upcoming appointments, since I was used to having my afternoons free for doctor visits. I moved my next acupuncture appointment to the morning.

At my second acupuncture appointment, Abby asked me to come into her office for a few minutes to talk to me. She said that she wanted me to come in twice a week for treatment, and that there were also some supplements that she wanted me to take that should help with my digestion and my immune system. She explained that normally she charges $35 per visit, and the supplements would come at an additional cost. To help me out, though, she said she was only going to charge me $35 per week, and that would include two office visits and any supplements that she gave me.

At first I thought I must be misunderstanding her, but I wasn't. She was going to give me two office visits per week for the price of one, and throw in the supplements for free. She seemed to genuinely want to help me, and my well-being was more important to her than making a buck. It filled me with so much hope and happiness to know that there were still people like that in the world after everything I had been through.

Working the afternoon/evening shift at 13 WHAM was an interesting change of pace. It really was a reversal of what I was used to, and not just in terms of the hours I was working. On the morning shift, we basically had a skeleton crew running the five a.m. news, and there were a lot more people in the building—producers, reporters, photographers, managers, sales/marketing, etc.—after nine a.m. On the evening shift, there was a full house there leading up to the five p.m. news and a skeleton crew by the time we got to the eleven p.m. newscast.

For this week of training, I came in at three p.m. and the director, AD, and I would get a list of the stories for the six o'clock news that needed BAM graphics. The BAM was the huge screen that the anchors stood in front of. It either stood for Behind

Anchor Monitor or Big Ass Monitor, depending on who you asked. We would then spend some time finding images on the web and putting them into templates to display in the BAM.

At around 5:30 p.m., we would get printed scripts from the producer. Each story that the anchor would read was on its own separate page. We would go through the stack of scripts and mark each one with notes so that we would be well prepared for when we were live on the air.

Directing was very fast-paced and exciting. I honestly found it thrilling. In addition to the novelty of it, this shift was easier on me physically. My symptoms tended to be worse in the morning and level off throughout the day. By the time I got to work at three p.m., I was not rushing to the restroom nearly as often as I was when I went in at 3:30 a.m. Being able to actually sleep in every morning was incredible.

The biggest drawback was the fact that Amanda and I were like ships passing in the night. By the time I got home at midnight, she would be asleep, and by the time I got up, she would be at work. We did not see each other at all that week.

I didn't get too used to it. After a week of training on the evening shift, I was right back to the 3:30 a.m. morning shift.

A couple of months had gone by since I started the Humira and the acupuncture, and I still was not seeing much relief. I ended up deciding not to continue with acupuncture. Even though Abby was giving me a discount, it was still $35 I was having to come up with every week on top of all of my other expenses, and it was time out of my day to drive there and back for treatment when all I wanted to do when I wasn't at work was curl up under a blanket at home. Most of all, it just didn't seem to be making any real difference with my symptoms.

By the end of March, Dr. Griswold had added the 6-MP, or mercaptopurine, to my treatment, which was one of the meds he had mentioned at the appointment where we first talked about Humira, the one that took a few months to build up in your system before it had any real effect. I guess at this point he figured we might as well throw it into the mix and see if it stuck. He also gave me a standing order for bloodwork, because 6-MP can lower your white blood cell count and increase your risk of infection, and it can also potentially cause inflammation of the liver. Routine blood tests every six weeks would ensure that this new med wasn't causing me any harm in those other areas.

In March, I got this email from my dad after I had stopped over to see him and my mom. He wrote to me from work.

Hi Russ,

It was good to see you yesterday. You are on my mind all the time. I hope you find the strength to deal with all you are going through. I feel strongly that things will improve for you soon, if you can hang in there. Mema said to remind you that you come from tough stock!

Remember you have a support network that cares about you very much. I know that thinking of that has helped me with my own health problems. Whenever I'm feeling good, I thank God for that period of time, no matter how short it is.

I'm so glad you have Amanda there for you. Focus your free time on her, and comics, and good movies/TV. Speaking of TV, the winner on Jeopardy last night is a huge comic book collector!

Well, gotta finish up some work before I go.

Hope to see you soon.

Love,

Dad

Focusing my free time on fun things seemed easier said than done. I felt so drained all the time that it was like I just didn't have the energy for them. Going out to the comic book store to grab the latest issues of Superman, Batman, and Spider-Man used to be something I loved. Now it seemed like too much effort. I just wasn't sure I was up for it. I didn't know at the time that losing interest in things you used to enjoy is a classic sign of depression.

I thought about what my dad said about being thankful for every minute that I felt good. When was the last time that I really had?

I knew my parents were worried about me all the time, and this was without them fully understanding how bad things were getting. I didn't want them to know how rough things were or how burnt out I felt almost all the time.

Chapter Sixteen

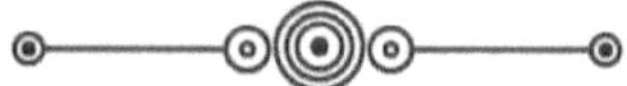

Earlier in 2008, Amanda's best friend Amber had mentioned that her boyfriend, Nick, had a good friend named Jared who also had Crohn's disease. Jared had been through a lot, and he was very open in talking about his struggles with Crohn's. Nick and Amber had mentioned to him that I had been diagnosed with it and wondered if maybe Jared would be open to reaching out to me so that we could connect and compare notes. Jared said he would be happy to talk to me and passed along his email address.

Jared and I emailed back and forth a couple of times. With my crazy work schedule and early bedtime, it took a little while for us to sync up for a phone call. Plus, I was a little hesitant to talk to him. My battle with Crohn's was still something that I kept to myself. The idea of commiserating with someone else who had shared the struggle was something I wanted to be able to do, but the walls that I had put up were hard to bring down.

One day in April, I was having a particularly bad day with my symptoms. The pain, frequency, and difficulty of my bowel movements prompted me to do a full day of eating absolutely nothing, so as to not put anything else into my battered and beaten digestive tract. I still took my Pentasa and prednisone, of course, but other than that, I didn't put anything else into my body all day besides water. I needed to talk to someone about this. I emailed Jared and asked if we could find time to chat.

Jared and I finally found time to connect for a phone call. He was a super nice, super friendly guy who was open to talking candidly about his own Crohn's story. It was the first time I'd ever talked directly with someone else who had the same disease as me.

Jared said that he had received a considerable amount of relief from his symptoms five years earlier, when he'd had surgery to remove a few inches of his small intestine. They had been able to locate where most of his inflammation was, and just go in and simply remove it. He had remained on steroids for a few months later, then slowly tapered off of them. He had been doing much better ever since, although he still took 6-MP as a maintenance drug to keep the inflammation from coming back.

With Crohn's disease, surgery is not a cure. The inflammation can, and often does, eventually return in another part of the digestive tract. However, the surgery can buy you years of relief before that happens. Jared said that, with the exception of popcorn and seeds, he was at a point where he could eat pretty much whatever he wanted. For someone like me, who had just gone a whole day eating absolutely nothing because my symptoms were so bad, that sounded like an absolute dream. Could this surgery be something that could work for me? I don't think anyone had ever felt so hopeful that maybe he could have some of his intestines cut out.

That was my first real conversation with someone else with Crohn's, but it wouldn't be my last. In fact, it would not even be my last in that same week. Amanda and I found a Crohn's and Colitis Support Group which was held at a local hospital. The group met six times a year; three Wednesdays in the spring and three Wednesdays in the fall. It met from seven p.m. to nine p.m., which was definitely past my bedtime. I was a little apprehensive about attending something that late, but I figured it would be good for me.

I was also, as usual, just nervous about being out in public, in a room with other people. Anytime I needed to be in a set place for a set length of time, I got so worried about the potential need to run out and find a bathroom. In this case, I'd be in a room with other people who had Crohn's or colitis and knew the struggle. That should have made it better, but in a way it made it worse. If I had to leave the room, of course they would all know what was happening. I was definitely overthinking things, but this is what was playing out in my mind as Amanda and I drove to the meeting.

The meeting was in a small conference room upstairs at the hospital. It was led by Brian and Betty, a married couple who both had Crohn's disease. Besides me and Amanda, there were about six or seven other people there. Betty set a few ground rules at the start of the meeting: no one was allowed to say the names of any doctors that they were seeing, and while you could mention medications that you were taking, you were not allowed to say what dose you were on.

Everyone went around the table, one at a time, giving an update on how they were doing. Everyone except me and Amanda had been to the group before. One of the women in the group had been taking part in a clinical trial for Crohn's disease that involved stem cells. I actually recognized her from a story about it that had been in the local newspaper.

When it got to be my turn, I shared my story of having been diagnosed with Crohn's about two years earlier.

"Oh, so not that long ago," Betty commented.

As I looked around the room, I noted that I was definitely the youngest person there. That scared me. How long was I going to have to live with this disease?

"It sure feels like a long time," I said.

Everyone nodded. They understood. Two years of feeling miserable all the time can feel like an eternity.

I talked about being on Pentasa and the prednisone yo-yo, and how I hated how the steroid made me feel. I talked about working two jobs and having to run to the bathroom all the time. I talked about Humira, and how I'd been able to get into the prescription assistance program for it. The others had not heard of the MyHumira program, so Betty made a note of it so she could suggest it to others. I even talked about how I'd talked to Jared a couple days ago, and that he'd had some success from having surgery. I threw it out there to kind of put the feelers out. Would anyone else in this room recommend the surgical option?

As a matter of fact, yes, the couple said they knew lots of people who had come to the group who had gotten years of relief from their Crohn's symptoms after having resection surgery. It was like Jared had said, they basically just cut out the section of your intestine where the inflammation is, and then reattach the pieces.

Brian shared his own story. He'd had surgery to have his entire colon and rectum removed, and he now had an ostomy bag. He was very comfortable talking about it. Here was this guy talking about how he has an ostomy bag and how much better his quality of life had been since he'd gotten it. It was crazy to me how open everyone was to talking about everything. It made me feel a lot less alone.

But the idea of having an ostomy bag terrified me. Having shit come out of my stomach and go into a bag for the rest of my life? I couldn't imagine it. I hoped that maybe I could get the resection surgery done like Jared had, just have the problematic part of my guts removed and everything else neatly put back together. Even if it only got me a few years of relief, that was a lot better than the zero relief I was getting now.

We continued to go around the table sharing our stories and updates. Amanda was to my left, so technically that made her next. They asked her if she wanted to share anything with the group.

"Hi, I'm Amanda, I'm Russ's fiancée. I don't have Crohn's disease," she said. Everyone gave a small laugh. There was a pause. And then, thoughtfully, Amanda added, "But sometimes I feel like I do."

I turned and looked at her in surprise. I didn't know what she meant by that. I had no idea she was going to say that, and truthfully until that moment, I don't think she did either.

"Russ's diet is so limited. We have to be so careful about what he eats. And because there are a lot of foods he can't have, I don't usually have them either. We don't go out much anymore, to restaurants or to go do anything fun. We always have to be conscious of where the bathrooms are. If we go for a walk, we have to make sure we don't go too far from our apartment in case he has to rush back. I just… I feel like I have Crohn's, too, sometimes."

I never knew she felt that way. I had not thought about how much my limitations had also become her limitations. Sure, she didn't have the inflammation and physical pain that I did. But all the lifestyle changes that came with trying to accommodate that had become her lifestyle changes as well. I grabbed her hand and squeezed it tight. We were in this together. I loved her for that, but I also hated what I had pulled her into. Maybe instead of her lifting me up, I was weighing her down.

Before we left the meeting that night, Betty gave me her email address. She told me to send her an email so she'd have mine, and she would send me the schedule for the rest of the meetings for the year.

The meeting ended. I was home and in bed around ten. I was back at work at 13 WHAM at 3:30 a.m.

The next evening was a really bad one for me. I was a huge fan of the TV show *Smallville*, the chronicles of a young Clark Kent, which aired on the CW. There was a new episode airing that night, titled "Descent." The internet was abuzz about the fact that this would be a pivotal episode in the character development of Michael Rosenbaum's Lex Luthor and his journey on the road to full-fledged villainy. I was so keen to watch it that, even though I had just stayed up late for the support group the night before, I was going to stay up again and watch the episode.

At least, that was what I had planned.

I got hit with a really intense, painful series of cramps that had me glued to the toilet for well over an hour that evening. I missed the whole episode. I had recorded it so I could watch it on the DVR, but by the time I was able to pull myself off the bowl it was so late I decided to just call it a night. The episode I had been looking forward to would have to wait for the next day. I was crushed. It wasn't so much that I had to wait to watch that episode, per se. It was the fact that my quality of life had gotten so bad that even watching a TV show at home was a pleasure that I was not guaranteed.

At my next follow-up with Dr. Griswold, I brought up the surgical option. I explained that even with the Humira, my symptoms were still really bad, and I'd been having a lot more bad days than good. Ever since I was in the hospital back in September, I really hadn't had my symptoms under control. I was having many painful bowel movements every single day, and that was with me eating a bland diet of mainly toast, chicken, chicken soup, and scrambled eggs. I needed to know what our next option was, and I asked if the surgery might be it.

He said that it was something that we could talk about, but that he wanted to do a couple of tests first: an upper GI series with small bowel follow-through, and another colonoscopy, since I hadn't had one since first being diagnosed back in Virginia. Before we could consider the surgical option, we needed to get a handle on exactly where my inflammation currently was. If it was mostly in the small bowel and terminal ilium, then I might do well with surgery. If the inflammation was extensive throughout my whole small bowel, or if it was in my colon/large intestine, then that was not something we would treat with surgery. This all made sense to me.

The upper GI series with small bowel follow-through was done at the hospital. This is a test to see if there's any inflammation or obstruction in the part of your digestive tract that includes your esophagus, stomach, and the first part of your small intestine. Since Crohn's disease can manifest in any part of your digestive system, Dr. Griswold wanted to make sure that there weren't any issues there. The test consists of drinking a special liquid containing barium that basically coats your guts and provides a high level of contrast when an x-ray is taken, making it easy to spot ulcers, polyps, or other issues or obstructions.

When I arrived at the imaging center, they gave me a large Styrofoam cup with a lid and a straw and told me that I needed to drink it. This was the barium. It didn't taste terrible, but it sure didn't taste great. It was thick and had kind of a chalky texture. I've heard of it being compared to a milkshake before, but that's being generous. The taste wasn't the hard part. Remember how I said I got uncomfortable at the thought of being in a room with people and knowing that it would be very obvious or visible if I had to leave to go to the bathroom? Being in a waiting room and drinking something that was going to have an unknown effect on my sensitive GI system, all while knowing I could be called by a technician at any time, also made me really anxious.

Eventually they called me back and had me go behind a small curtained-off area and change out of my clothes and into a gown. Then they took me back into an exam room and had me lie down on a table.

The x-ray is taken with a specific kind of machine called a fluoroscope. While you lie stationary on the table, the fluoroscope is moved up or down by the technician to get it positioned over the right spot. It takes kind of a "movie" x-ray as well as still images, to show how the barium contrast liquid is moving through your digestive tract. It only took a few minutes for them to get the images that they needed from me. A few times, they asked me to hold my breath while they took the x-rays.

It was definitely quick, easy, and painless, but I was a bundle of nerves the whole time. I couldn't help but think: What if this liquid I just drank hits me wrong and I need to use the bathroom right away? Can I just get up and leave? I was mortified at the thought of asking them to stop taking x-rays so I could get up and run to the bathroom. Fortunately that did not happen. Before long, I was changing back out of my gown and into my clothes.

I didn't really feel the effects of the barium on my digestive system until the afternoon. For a couple of hours, I had very painful, straining bowel movements that felt like my bowels were trying to wring themselves out like a used dishcloth. The stuff coming out of me was white and milky.

My colonoscopy was scheduled for just three days later, which meant that I'd be engaging in another round of "prep." Dr. Griswold prescribed me something a little different for this one: MoviPrep. I love that name. Sounds like we're just getting ready to watch a movie, right? How fun. It cost me $44.79 at the Wegmans pharmacy. Dr. Griswold had me precede it with two Dulcolax tablets, which is a laxative that you can purchase over the counter.

My experience with MoviPrep was quite a bit different than with GoLYTELY. If you'll recall, the GoLYTELY kicked in pretty much right around the one-hour mark of drinking it. With the MoviPrep, I had been drinking it for over two hours and was actually closing in on my last couple of glasses of it and nothing had taken effect yet. I was starting to get worried that maybe it wasn't going to work for some reason. Also, the MoviPrep was a lot less palatable.

Then, after the seventh or eighth glass, I started feeling nauseous. With each subsequent glass, I wondered if I was going to puke. My stomach was not liking this stuff, but instead of making me crap my brains out, it was making me want to hurl. What if I vomited the stuff up? Would it still work? What was I supposed to do? What if I just stopped drinking it? Had I taken enough of it to do the trick? Drinking the GoLYTELY had been a chore, but the MoviPrep was requiring some serious effort. I had to literally choke down the last couple of glasses, gagging and struggling not to vomit after each gulp.

When the MoviPrep finally hit, it hit hard. I was in the bathroom all night. After the first few hours of nonstop defecating, I tried to go to bed, but it was pointless. I'd be back up and sprinting to the bathroom again before I could fall asleep.

My mom came to the apartment bright and early the next morning, as she and Amanda were both going to come to the appointment with me. We were supposed to arrive at the Westfall Surgery Center in Brighton at 7:00 a.m. for a 7:30 a.m. procedure. When my mom got to our apartment at about 6:20 a.m., I was still in the bathroom. There was still stuff coming out of me. Not a lot, but enough that I didn't feel like I could leave the bathroom. I resolved that if I ever had to get another colonoscopy, I would start the prep much earlier.

Once they finally got me out the door, the actual procedure was pretty unmemorable. Just like the first time, they put me right to sleep. Though the fact that I hadn't slept a wink the night before probably helped. I was out like a light through the entire procedure.

After the colonoscopy, my mom and Amanda and I went out to IHOP for breakfast. Normally going out to restaurants to eat terrified me, but I was feeling so relaxed from the sedatives I basically felt like I was drunk, and I wanted pancakes, damn it! I was so glad that the procedure was over, and the meds had me feeling so good that my usual fear of eating was gone. I shoved pancakes into my mouth like they were going out of style.

Once they got me back home to the apartment, I went to bed and slept the rest of the day away.

My follow-up with Dr. Griswold to discuss the results of both tests was one week later. My mom came with me to the appointment.

"Your upper GI was perfect. Everything is normal there. No inflammation, no obstruction, everything on the upper GI looks good," Dr. Griswold explained. So that meant my trachea, stomach, and the first part of my small bowel were all free and clear.

"There was no evidence of ulceration in your small bowel or terminal ilium, either," Dr. Griswold continued. This surprised me because I specifically remembered Dr. Harvey saying I did have ulcers in my terminal ilium when he first diagnosed me. "What we do see is inflammation through the descending colon. There's no obstruction there, but there is a lot of inflammation. The disease is in your rectum, near the anal sphincter. This means that a resection surgery like we had discussed would not apply here. Treating your disease with surgery would entail removing your colon and rectum. You'd have an ostomy bag for the rest of your life. It doesn't make sense to do something that extreme here."

I was crushed. I had gone into this appointment thinking Dr. Griswold would say I'd be a good candidate for the same surgery as Jared, and that I'd be on my way to years of relief from what I'd been going through. Turns out, it was not going to be that simple. I felt like Charlie Brown, once again having the football pulled away just when I was sure I was going to kick it this time.

"What we need to do is treat the inflammation," Dr. Griswold continued. "I'm going to prescribe you two antibiotics. Xifaxan fights bacterial infections specifically in the intestines. Ciprofloxacin also fights bacteria that can aggravate Crohn's symptoms. I'm also going to add a hydrocortisone retention enema. This is a corticosteroid that's taken rectally that reduces inflammation in the colon and rectum."

So instead of the easy answer of just cutting this disease out of me, I had three more things to add to my regimen. I would now be taking Pentasa, prednisone, Humira, 6-MP, ciprofloxacin, Xifaxan, and a hydrocortisone enema. My kitchen counter was starting to look like a pharmacy, and I was feeling more discouraged than ever.

Chapter Seventeen

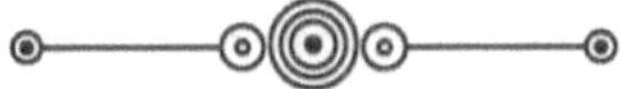

In June 2008, Dr. Griswold told me about another angle he wanted to pursue. He wanted me to take a test to see if I was lactose intolerant, in case that might be an underlying sensitivity that was exacerbating my symptoms. He sent me to Rochester General Hospital for the test. Amanda came with me.

They took a sample of my blood at the start of the test. Then they had me drink a liquid that contained lactose. They took additional blood samples about every twenty minutes or so, for a couple of hours. The test checks the glucose levels in your blood. If you are not lactose intolerant, your body breaks lactose down into glucose, and the glucose levels in your blood rise after you drink the lactose. If you are lactose intolerant, your body doesn't break down the lactose the way that it should, and the glucose levels in your blood do not rise by much.

I imagine another way they could assess your lactose intolerance would be seeing if you spend most of the test in agony in the bathroom after drinking the lactose, which I did.

Fortunately there was a bathroom right off of the waiting room where I was sitting between each blood draw. I was getting hit pretty quickly with symptoms very similar to when I passed the rest of the barium contrast stuff after my upper GI series. It was a loose, appropriately "milky" consistency.

I'd be on the toilet and I would hear the technician call my name for the next blood draw. I'd hear Amanda say, "He's in the bathroom." I'd finish up as quickly as I could, then come out. The technician would be gone, so I'd have to sheepishly go up to the check-in window and say, "Hi, they called my name. I was in the bathroom."

By the time the test was over, the technician was actually apologizing to me for putting me through this. "I obviously can't say this officially until the test results are in, but I think it's safe to say you're lactose intolerant," he commented while taking my last blood draw, having seen how much time I'd been spending in the bathroom.

When I saw Dr. Griswold again the following week to discuss the results, he said, "You're *very* lactose intolerant! Like, holy shit are you lactose intolerant!" If a doctor says "holy shit" while looking at your test results, you know you've really shown them something.

Dr. Griswold changed my prednisone prescription to the liquid form, because the pills actually contained lactose and the liquid did not. He advised me to completely cut milk and anything containing lactose out of my diet for now. Eventually we could try re-introducing it alongside some enzymes that assist with lactose digestion, but for now, he wanted me to omit it completely and monitor my symptoms.

On Wednesdays, Amanda worked late because she had music therapy sessions in Buffalo. I usually went over to my parents' house on Wednesdays to visit, have dinner, and throw in a load of laundry. Now that I had been established as lactose intolerant, the list of things I could have for dinner was growing even smaller.

One time when I was over there, my mom was making sure that something she was making for dinner did not have any dairy ingredients. She double-checked the recipe and said, "I just want to make sure this is kosher." By that, she just meant make sure it was "all right" for me to eat. But my grandma had just walked in the room, and she exclaimed, "Now Russ is on a kosher diet?"

I had to laugh. Who knows, maybe that would be next!

By this time, I was starting to really struggle financially. My insurance had a $500 deductible, which meant that I was paying completely out of pocket for all of these tests and all of my office visits with Dr. Griswold the first part of the year, on top of all the medications. I was so desperate to make my Pentasa last longer between each refill that I wasn't taking it properly.

When I was starting to get low, I'd take just one pill instead of two, or I'd skip doses, just to stretch out the time before I had to fill it again. I reasoned that having at least some of it in my system had to be better than having none. Amanda and I were trying to plan a wedding, paying rent on an apartment, paying student loans, paying the electric bill, the cable bill, the cell phone bill, and all the while my medical bills were piling up.

Some of the medical bills would come with a due date of a few weeks out. Others, usually the lab tests, would come with "due upon receipt" as the due date. If it had a date a few weeks out, I would plan accordingly and try my best to mail in a check to pay it on time. Anything that showed up with "due upon receipt" made me irrationally angry and I wouldn't pay it. It seemed to offend me somehow that they were saying "we need this money immediately," and I wouldn't send them anything.

Eventually I'd get a second notice, and then usually a third before I finally got a notice that it was about to be sent to a collection agency. Once they started threatening me with the collection agency, I'd send a check. For example, in July I still owed $93.64 for that upper GI series from back in April. I never told Amanda or my parents about this. I didn't want them to worry, and I didn't want to burden them with any of it. I was beyond frustrated to be working seven days a week, only to have most of my money going to doctors, tests, and medicines that were not making me better.

In the summer, we had a going away party at our apartment for our friends Nick and Amber who were moving to Albany. They were the ones who had connected me with Jared. Amanda was cleaning the apartment before the party, and I offered to run out to Wegmans to get a bunch of snacks. Even though I knew I would not be able to eat any of the snacks myself, I wanted to contribute to the party by getting a bunch of goodies for everyone else to enjoy.

While I was out, I got violently sick. Wegmans was only a few minutes' drive from our apartment, but I had to stop at McDonald's to use the bathroom before I even got to Wegmans. Then I had to run to the bathroom again when I got to Wegmans.

As I sat in the stall, I thought about the fact that in about an hour, our apartment would be full of people, and instead of having fun, I would be hoping that the bathrooms weren't occupied if I needed one in a hurry. I'd be watching everyone else enjoy pizza and chips and wine and pop and a veggie tray and Rice Krispies treats while I would be eating absolutely nothing and just hoping to not get sick.

A bunch of our friends from the party spent the night. The next morning, everyone was getting up early and going on a wine tour. I was not up for that. I couldn't handle the idea of leaving the house or being in a vehicle on a long drive with everyone, let alone the fact that I wouldn't be able to drink any of the wine anyway. I stayed in bed while everyone was getting ready to leave. I didn't want to face everyone or have anyone try to talk me into coming or feel bad for me because I wasn't going.

As I was lying in bed, I suddenly needed to go to the bathroom. I could hear through the closed bedroom door that everyone was about to leave. They were by the front door putting on shoes, gathering up purses. I knew that any minute, maybe even any second, everyone would be gone and I would be alone in the apartment. I didn't want everyone to see me run out of the bedroom into the bathroom. I just didn't want everyone to have one more reminder of me and my disease and that I wasn't coming on the wine tour. If I could just hold out, maybe even just thirty more seconds, I'd hear the front door close and I could sprint to the bathroom and no one would know…

I shit my pants in bed, so violently that I also pissed myself. That's right. In those last few seconds that I was waiting for my fiancée and her friends to leave the apartment, I was in the bedroom, in bed, and shit and pissed myself because I didn't want everyone to see me run to the bathroom. And as soon as I had completely evacuated everything from my bladder and bowels, I heard the front door shut and the apartment was empty.

Now I got to spend my morning of solitude doing cleanup on the sheets I'd just soiled. Fortunately, the fecal matter had all stayed in my pants and didn't get on the sheets at all, but I had still wet them. So, after showering and changing my clothes, I gathered the sheets off the bed and carried them out across the parking lot to the apartment complex laundry room. I had them washed, dried, and returned to the bed before anyone got home. I never told Amanda that this happened.

One day, I was on my way home from working the morning shift at 13 WHAM, and on a whim I decided I would stop at the library in Chili. They had a great selection of graphic novels, and I thought maybe I could check out something fun to read to take my mind off how miserable I was feeling.

I was looking through the graphic novels when suddenly I felt very urgently sick and needed to use the bathroom. I made my way as quickly as I could to the bathroom without running, only to find that it was locked. Apparently I needed to get a key from the front desk. I didn't have time for that. I physically would not have been able to make it to the desk, ask for the key, get it, and make it back to the bathroom.

While I stood there silently shuddering with my eyes closed, I defecated in my pants, standing right outside of the locked bathroom. I sadly shuffled out of the library, no graphic novel in hand, and got awkwardly back into my car. Because my pants were full of shit, I couldn't sit down on the seat. I suspended myself up off of the seat with my right hand and left foot, just like when I drove myself to the walk-in clinic in Virginia when I had that cyst.

I couldn't keep living like this. Something needed to change. I liked Dr. Griswold, but I felt like he was out of ideas on how to make me better.

It was time for me to get another opinion.

Chapter Eighteen

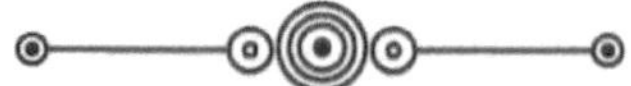

My mom knew I was thinking of switching doctors, and she wanted to make sure I got connected with someone who would be proactive and really work on getting me feeling better. She emailed the president of the local chapter of the Crohn's and Colitis Foundation of America, asking if he could put us in touch with anyone who could recommend a gastroenterologist who was "good" with Crohn's patients.

He wrote back and said that he would be glad to speak with me, but only as a fellow Crohn's patient and not as an affiliate of the CCFA. Again, much like with the support group, the CCFA was not allowed to recommend one doctor over another. But he was willing to speak with me "off the record" as long as it was clear we were discussing his personal experiences and he was not making any kind of official endorsements on behalf of the CCFA. I thought that was really cool. My mom passed along his email, which included his home phone number.

I gave him a call. He was a very nice, friendly guy, sympathetic to my situation since he was a Crohn's patient himself; he knew the struggles I was going through and could relate to the kind of state that I was in. He made it clear that what he was about to say was not the CCFA giving this advice, but just him, as a fellow patient. If the CCFA was to recommend one doctor over another, they would run the risk of offending or alienating the doctors they were not recommending. I told him I completely understood.

With that disclaimer out of the way, he asked me who I was currently seeing for a GI doc. I told him Dr. Griswold.

"I consider myself to be fairly 'plugged in' to which GI doctors in the Rochester area are good for Crohn's, and I have to tell you, I have never heard of Dr. Griswold before," he said.

This just reinforced my theory that Dr. Griswold was out of his depth when it came to trying to help my case.

"I can tell you who I go to," he continued. "My doctor that I have seen for many years is Dr. Shreck at Strong Memorial Hospital. I've always been very happy with him; he's very smart and knows his stuff. I've heard some people say that they have trouble understanding him or have trouble communicating with him, but I've never found that to be a problem at all myself. I also know Dr. Calvin at Rochester General Hospital very well, he is an excellent GI for Crohn's disease as well, to give you a second name. Overall, though, I'd recommend going to a research institution like Strong Memorial Hospital. Getting in with a digestive specialist there, like Dr. Shreck, is going to mean they are up on the latest and best treatments."

I was sold. The fact that this guy had personally been seeing Dr. Shreck and had success with him was enough for me, and the point he made about Strong being a research hospital and being up on the latest and greatest stuff in the field was icing on the cake.

I made a call and scheduled an appointment to see Dr. Shreck for a second opinion on my treatment.

In late July 2008, Amanda and I went to see Dr. Shreck for the first time. There was a whole group of medical buildings in the Clinton Crossings area of Rochester. It took a little bit of time and effort to find the right building as we drove past a cluster of nearly identical buildings, but something about it made it seem like this was the real deal. Like you had reached the hub of so much medical knowledge.

Dr. Griswold's office had been in just one solitary building that had other offices in it that were not even all medical people. Not that that is any indication of the quality of care you are going to receive, but something about Dr. Shreck being part of this huge, expansive medical community made it seem like he was more legit.

We eventually found the right building and signed in at the reception desk. We also noticed that there were several doctors in the practice, not just Dr. Shreck. The waiting room was huge, and people were all waiting to see one of a number of different GI specialists. It made the experience feel more "big leagues."

When we got called back to the exam room, we didn't see Dr. Shreck right away. The first person who came back to talk to us was a nurse practitioner named Lorraine. She was very pleasant. She sat down with us and asked about my history with Crohn's and what brought us to see Dr. Shreck.

I gave her the whole story. That I'd first started experiencing symptoms in 2005 and that I was diagnosed with Crohn's in March of 2006. I told her my medication regimen and that I'd recently discovered I was lactose intolerant. I told her I was still having many loose, urgent bowel movements every day and pain in my abdomen and that I wanted to see Dr. Shreck because I wanted a second opinion as I didn't feel like my symptoms were under control.

The whole time I was talking, she listened carefully and took notes on everything. She took her time to get every detail. She asked me questions, like how often there was blood in my stool (occasionally), and if I ever woke up in the middle of the night with the need to run to the bathroom (rarely), and if I ever had any rashes, fevers, sores in my mouth (no, no, and no). She asked about my family history and whether anyone else in my family had Crohn's or any other GI diseases (not that I know of).

After we finished going over everything, she said she was going to step out and get Dr. Shreck. I wondered if I was going to have to repeat everything to him.

But when Lorraine came back in with the doctor, she gave him a superfast recap of everything that we had just talked about. She was looking at her notes and speaking very quickly but clearly. This was obviously the routine for them.

Dr. Shreck sat down on a chair in the corner of the exam room. He listened as she recited the list of medications that I was on.

He looked at me. "You have tried Remicade?" he asked.

"No, sir," I said. "We skipped over that one. Dr. Griswold thought Humira would be better." All I could think of was the infusions and the mouse-human thing. I hoped he would not say I should try that.

He rubbed his chin and thought for a moment. "The lactose tolerance test you had done, why did they do a blood test?"

"To… see if I was lactose intolerant," I said, completely missing the point of the question. "Dr. Griswold thought that that might be contributing to my symptoms, so we—"

"No, no," he said, waving his hand and shaking his head. "Why did they do a blood test? For lactose intolerance, the breath test is much more reliable."

"Oh," I said. "I didn't know that. I'm not sure."

"Okay. We will recheck this. We will do a breath test this time. I would also like to do a stool study, a C-difficile, a fecal lactoferrin and O and P." Lorraine was scribbling all of this down as he spoke. "We will also want to check a CBC, Chem-14, and CRP level as well. I would also like to do another colonoscopy."

Lorraine mentioned that I had just had one in April, and she also told Dr. Shreck about the CT scan that I was scheduled to have done the next day, which Dr. Griswold had ordered for me.

"That's fine, proceed with the CT scan," Dr. Shreck said. "But I do still want to do another colonoscopy as well. I am also going to alter your medications. Discontinue the retention enema, we will get you a Cortifoam enema to take in the evening and a Canasa suppository to take in the morning. These will treat the rectal inflammation. You know how to take a suppository?"

"I… I'm pretty sure I do," I said, not particularly looking forward to it.

"After the colonoscopy, we will work on getting you off the prednisone." He was already standing up and walking out of the office as Lorraine worked to finish writing all of this down. On his way out the door, he looked at me and nodded. "We will get you better." Then he left the room.

On the drive home, Amanda commented on that last remark. "I really like how he said, 'We will get you better.' That's what we need. Someone who is committed to getting you healthy again, Russ!"

I liked his confidence as well, but my head was spinning. I hadn't expected Dr. Shreck to change my meds. I kind of figured that when you got a second opinion, they just gave you some additional ideas of things that you could try, and then you went back to your regular doctor and talked about them. Maybe that is how it works sometimes. I certainly wasn't expecting to walk out of there with a list of more tests that I was going to take, including a third colonoscopy—my second one for the year—and some new prescriptions to fill. Still, his parting words echoed in my ears. *We will get you better.* I sure hoped so.

My CT scan was the day after my appointment with Dr. Shreck, at the same place where I'd had the upper GI series. The process was very similar, at least from my perspective. I had to drink another cup of oral contrast, then wait about ninety minutes for it to work its way to my abdomen before they called me back for the scan.

This procedure had an added bonus of an IV as well, so they could intravenously administer a second type of contrast called Optiray 350. As they were about to start the IV, they warned me that I would probably feel a sensation like a warm rush through my body that makes some patients feel like they have to go to the bathroom. Great, like I didn't already feel like that all the time.

I did feel a warm sort of tingling through my arm and then through the rest of my body that I actually thought was kind of pleasant and relaxing. It did not make me feel like I had to go to the bathroom, at least not any more than usual… but since that thought had been put in my head, all I could think about was what if I had to go to the bathroom during this process? It was only going to take a few minutes, right?

Much like the upper GI scan, I laid down on a table. The scanner for the CT scan looked kind of like a big donut, and the table I laid on moved me back and forth through the hole of the donut. On the side of the donut, there were little smiley-face pictures that would light up, one that was holding his breath and one that was just normal looking. As the technician was about to start taking a scan, a prerecorded voice would say "Hold your breath" and the holding-his-breath smiley face would light up. I would move through the donut and it would take some pictures. Then the voice would say "Breathe normally" and the non-holding-his-breath smiley face would light up.

I tried to just relax as much as I could and focus on my breathing. Even so, that little voice of worry was still in the back of my head, trying to plan what I would do if I suddenly had to go to the bathroom. Being as we were right in the middle of the scan, I did not feel like I could reasonably say "Hey, can we stop for a second? I have to use the bathroom." So what would I do? Had anyone ever shit themselves during a CT scan? If that happened to me right now, I couldn't possibly be the first, right? These were the kinds of things I was thinking about.

The scans really only took a couple of minutes, with a few rounds of holding my breath and letting it out. Before I knew it, the technician was telling me that I could get up and go back and get dressed. As I was leaving, they advised me to drink plenty of fluids for the next twenty-four hours to help flush the contrast out of my body. The results of the scan would be sent to Dr. Griswold and Dr. Shreck. At this point, I couldn't wait to get home and just drink some water and relax.

The next morning, I was finishing up my early-morning shift at 13 WHAM when I missed a call on my cell from Dr. Shreck. As soon as I had a chance, I ran to the bathroom, both because I had to relieve myself and because I wanted a quiet place to listen to the voicemail he had left.

"Hello, Russell," Dr. Shreck said on the voicemail. "I have reviewed the results of your CT scan. There is actually very little inflammation present, some in your rectum and some in your left colon, but it is not serious. There is a large amount of stool in the right colon. Overall, I am not concerned by what I am seeing here."

I played the message a second time because I felt like I must be missing something. There was a large amount of stool present in the right colon? *Okay, so… what do we do about that? How do we get it so it's, like, out? You're not very concerned, but I am! What am I supposed to do?*

I also received a voicemail not too long after that from Dr. Griswold's office. This one was not so much commenting on the CT scan, but the fact that I was now essentially seeing two doctors. The message said that they understood that I had sought a second opinion from Dr. Shreck, and while of course they had no problem with me doing so, I would need to choose whether I was going to continue to see Dr. Griswold or switch over to Dr. Shreck's care.

I now had a big decision to make.

But before I could make that decision, I was going to talk to another doctor.

Chapter Nineteen

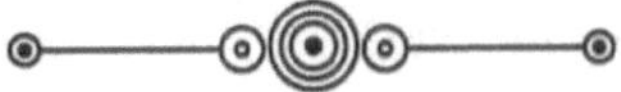

I was talking to my dad about the fact that I was wrestling with the idea of switching doctors. Did I stick with Dr. Griswold or make the jump to Dr. Shreck? My dad's response was, "Maybe it's time to talk to Doctor Bill."

Dr. Bill Valenti is an infectious disease specialist and a pioneer in the subject of HIV/AIDS treatment and research. He is the co-founder of Trillium Health, a leading LGBTQ+ healthcare provider in Rochester, New York. He is also my dad's cousin. (His cousin once removed, technically. Bill's father and my dad's grandmother were brother and sister.) Considering everything I had already been through, finding myself at this crossroads with my medical care was daunting. My dad thought that getting some advice from an experienced physician who was also a member of the family might help me with the next steps.

I was hesitant. I had only met Bill once before at a family reunion, and that was many years ago. Also, as we have established, talking about my health issues with anyone was not easy for me. Even though he was a doctor and a member of the family, I knew I would feel weird talking to him about what I was going through. Also, his specialty was infectious diseases, not Crohn's. What if he was not able to help me? I'd hate to bother him for no good reason.

That's how I felt almost all the time. That I would hate to be a bother. I was suffering every day and didn't want to bother anyone with that fact.

What I did not know at the time was that Mema and Pepa had already been filling Dr. Bill in on some of my struggles, and my dad had called and spoken to him as well. Dr. Bill said he would be glad to talk with me.

Since the conversation had already started, I figured I should probably be a part of it.

I began with an email.

Dear Dr. Bill,

This is Russ Dimino. My dad told me he called you about my health problems with my Crohn's disease, and he passed your e-mail address along to me.

Right now I am taking Pentasa (4000 mg/day), prednisone (15 mg/day), ciprofloxacin (1000 mg/day), 6-MP (50 mg/day), and Humira (40 mg every 2 weeks). Despite all these meds, I am still having considerable problems, including frequent, urgent, painful bowel movements every day. I am barely eating anything because it seems like everything I eat makes me sick and causes more pain.

I felt like my current gastroenterologist, Dr. Griswold, was running out of ideas of what to do for me. Nothing seemed to be helping. I had gotten the name of another GI in the area, and I went to him for a second opinion, to see if he had anything else to suggest. His name is Dr. Shreck and he is based at Strong Hospital. Since I was just going for a second opinion, I was surprised that he said he wanted to do a colonoscopy on me himself (I just had one done by Dr. Griswold in April), and he wanted to change my meds... he changed a hydrocortisone retention enema that I had been doing to a Cortifoam version and added a daily Canasa mesalamine suppository to treat the rectal inflammation.

Now I am in the position of having to choose between doctors. On the one hand, I have been going to Dr. Griswold for about a year now, and I like him and am comfortable with him, but I don't feel like we are getting anywhere with treating my disease, and I really do get the impression that he doesn't know what else to do at this point. On the other hand, Dr. Shreck comes recommended from another Crohn's patient, and I like that he is based at a research hospital like Strong. I think I probably should make the switch but I feel some hesitation about changing to a new doctor who I don't know as well.

I also just had a CT scan done, and Dr. Shreck looked at the results. He said there is a lot of stool in my right colon and inflammation in my rectum and left colon, but it's "not serious" and "nothing to worry about" at this time. While I am glad they didn't find anything serious, it's frustrating to be told "not to worry" when I am in pain all the time and feel lousy every day.

I guess I was just wondering if you can offer any insight or advice on my potentially switching doctors, or any other comments or thoughts that you might be able to share about the situation. Thanks for taking the time, I really look forward to hearing from you.

Thanks, Dr. Bill.

Russ

I had a reply from him about an hour and twenty minutes later.

Russ-

Have a few thoughts I can share. Working in Mexico City at the moment and will return to ROC late Tues eve, Aug 12.

Do you have any time during the day to discuss. You could come to my house or we could meet someplace convenient. Am in good shape in the AM, Aug 13-15.

In terms of changing docs...I have worked with both Griswold and Shreck a lot over the years. There is nothing wrong with changing docs to get a fresh start on things.

Let me know your availability and let's talk more on this. If you don't have time those days, we can do it on the phone or via email.

BV

He was in Mexico City and still took the time to shoot me a reply! Wow. My worry that I might be a bother melted away. It was a great feeling.

We wrote back and forth a couple of more times to try to figure out a time to sync up and talk. He had extended the offer that I could come over and meet with him at his house. This made me uncomfortable for the same reason that going anywhere always made me uncomfortable—I knew I would have to go to the bathroom. Meeting with Dr. Bill at his house and having to excuse myself, multiple times, to use his bathroom was something I just could not fathom doing. I used my crazy work schedule as an excuse and said that talking over the phone would be easier for me. We set aside time for a phone call.

We had a nice conversation. It was still hard for me to open up and talk about my symptoms; I had gotten so accustomed to hiding them and keeping them a secret. But it did feel good to talk to someone like Dr. Bill, who was very knowledgeable and also very kind and empathetic. He did not make me feel self-conscious at all. He just genuinely seemed to want to help steer me in the right direction.

"It's a complicated problem," Dr. Bill said. "It's good to get a fresh perspective on it every so often." It turns out, Dr. Bill had spent some time with Dr. Shreck many years ago when Dr. Bill was a resident rotating through the GI service at Genesee Hospital. He told me to mention him and give Dr. Shreck his regards.

He also encouraged me to see about getting into a clinical trial if possible. There was a lot being done in terms of new drugs and new treatments for Crohn's, and he said I should see about getting into one. Stem cells, LDN (low-dose naltrexone), and TYSABRI were a few that he mentioned. He said I should ask Dr. Shreck about some of these newer agents, and whether some of these more contemporary therapies might be something I could get access to and maybe find some relief there. He did add that many clinical trials had requirements regarding what drugs or treatments you had already tried, or things that needed to "fail" for you before you could be admitted into the trial. With everything I had tried so far, I found it hard to believe there would be anything I wouldn't qualify for!

He also advised me to "map out" where my treatment was headed with Dr. Shreck. "What is our time frame? What's the next step? How will we know if this is or isn't working? If it's not, what's next? If there is a clinical trial in my future, how do I get there?" This made a lot of sense to me but also seemed intimidating. I think because I had to keep telling myself that the magic cure-all answer was right around the corner. I had to believe that the next thing I tried was going to be "it." So even entertaining the notion of *how long will I try this, and then if that doesn't work, what's next?* seemed so daunting. Considering everything I had already been through, it was hard to accept that there might be a lot more road ahead of me yet.

Dr. Bill also suggested something that my parents had been encouraging me to do, and that was to speak with a dietician. With the very limited diet I was currently on, there was concern that I was not getting enough nutrition. I was reluctant to do this.

I was worried that a dietician would recommend something that would end up making my symptoms worse.

At this point, I was barely eating. I was surviving on eggs, toast, tuna fish, rice, boiled chicken, mashed potatoes, pretzels… I knew it was far from a balanced diet. I was afraid I would talk to a dietician and they would have me reintroduce foods that I was not ready for and could not handle. My very basic diet brought me at least some level of comfort because at least I was controlling it.

Toward the end of the call, I asked Dr. Bill if he thought I should officially make the jump and switch to Dr. Shreck's care. Dr. Bill replied simply, "Shreck is one of the best." He told me to keep in touch and let him know how things went.

It was nice to talk to him, and his advice made sense, but like I said, it was still intimidating. It felt like I was stuck on the side of Mount Everest and had just gotten assistance from an expert mountain climber. His guidance was invaluable, but I just wanted to be off the damn mountain already!

As the summer of 2008 was coming to an end, Amanda and I attended a festival in town with live music, food vendors, and fireworks. Doing things like this was really hard for me. Being at an outdoor festival with no immediate restroom access made me super anxious. I was also becoming self-conscious about my appearance. The fabled "moon face" that often comes with prednisone had taken effect by now—my cheeks were perpetually puffy and swollen, and I was now prone to breakouts of acne on my forehead. But even though my instinct was to hide myself away like the Phantom of the Opera, I was trying to find some kind of a balance so that Amanda and I could still have a life. She had loved fireworks ever since she was a kid. Her dad, a Vietnam veteran and a very patriotic man, would always take Amanda and her siblings to see fireworks shows on the Fourth of July. Now, as an adult, she never passed up a chance to see them if she could.

We found an open spot on a small hill that was close to a McDonald's, so I could run in and use the restroom if I needed to. It made me feel a little more at ease to have a plan. Amanda and I laid down on the grass, side by side, looking up at the sky.

As the night lit up with brilliant explosions of color, I glanced over at Amanda's face. Her smile was wide and her eyes were bright with excitement. I was glad we were there. Even though I spent most of my time wanting to withdraw from the world, I still needed to remember to live in it. I didn't want to miss moments like this.

Chapter Twenty

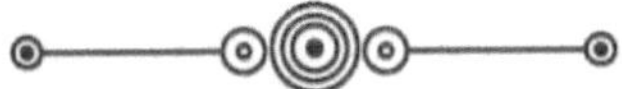

I made the decision to switch to Dr. Shreck. The next thing he wanted me to do was have the breath test done regarding my lactose intolerance. I was not really sure why I needed to do this. The blood test had shown Dr. Griswold that I was "holy shit" levels of lactose intolerant. Dr. Shreck said the breath test was more reliable. What was that going to do? Make him say "holy fuck"? I didn't really see the point of doing this when I was already just avoiding dairy, and that seemed simple enough.

But I wanted a good, clean start with Dr. Shreck, and I didn't feel like blowing off one of his first requests was going to get us off on the right foot. Despite me feeling that it was unnecessary, I went and had a breath lactose test done at the University of Rochester Medical Center.

The process was much the same as the blood test. I still had to drink a concoction with high amounts of lactose in it. But instead of me coming out of the bathroom every so often so they could take some of my blood, I came out of the bathroom every so often so I could breathe into a tube.

A couple of days later, I got a call from Dr. Shreck's office.

The results of my breath test said I was not lactose intolerant at all.

This made no sense.

I talked to my dad about it, and he was livid. He wanted to know how two tests could show two completely different things. He asked my permission to call Dr. Shreck's office and talk to him himself. I said go for it.

When my dad spoke with Dr. Shreck, the doctor again stated that the breath test is much more reliable than the blood test when it comes to determining lactose intolerance. When my dad asked why the tests would show different results, Dr. Shreck just kept reiterating that the breath test is more accurate, without really explaining how or why the blood test could have possibly shown the complete opposite result. He also said that because I have difficulty tolerating many foods due to my Crohn's disease, he recommended a low-residue diet and that I speak with a nutritionist. None of this really answered the question. I decided I would keep avoiding dairy anyway, even though now I was not really sure whether I was truly lactose intolerant or not.

I've mentioned a couple of times that Dr. Griswold and Dr. Shreck each had me doing some form of enema or another. Essentially, the point of the enema is to put a steroid right up into your rectum where the inflammation is, so it can work directly on that area. Think of it like putting a topical cream on a cut, only in this case the "cut" is way up inside your bum. What you have to do is either lie face down, propping your butt up into the air, or lie on your side. (Obviously, follow your doctor's instructions if you ever have to do this.) Then you gently insert the tip of a kind of squeeze-bottle up into your rectum and squeeze the steroid right up in there. The trick is you then need to retain it as long as possible. Ideally you can do it lying in bed, squirt the enema up there, and then go to sleep. This is what I would usually try to do, at least at first.

The problem was that the inflammation in my rectum was so bad that as soon as the steroid went in there, I felt the overwhelming urge to get it out, and get it out *now*. It burned, and I could feel my sphincter spasming and trying to push what I had just basted it with back out. I was lucky if I could hold it in for thirty seconds, maybe a minute, before I would have to sprint to the bathroom and let it all back out.

Eventually I stopped trying to do this in bed. I'd just lie down on the floor of our tiny little apartment bathroom, kind of curled up around the side of the toilet because there was not enough room for me to be fully prostrate, squirt the enema up into my anus, and then try to hold it in as long as I could. Sometimes I could only retain it for a few seconds. I'd try and try to clench and squeeze and bear down and keep it in as long as I could, but it was agony. It felt like I was pouring salt on a wound.

Amanda and I came to refer to this ridiculous process as "doing my thing," because I would let her know, "Hey, I'm going to go do my thing now." So yeah, "doing my thing" meant steroid enema up my ass.

At this time, I was still working the early shift at 13 WHAM, trying to get through each marathon of a morning in the studio without my symptoms getting the best of me.

I had my bathroom breaks down to a science. The show was timed very specifically. I knew the lengths of all the breaks by heart, so I could slip out to one of the bathrooms and know how quickly I had to relieve myself and be back in studio. Given the fact that I was spending most of my morning shift clenching my bowels shut and praying not to have an accident, even two minutes to run to the nearest restroom and get some fast relief was something I frequently took advantage of. The breaks were so routinely timed that if we were ever running behind schedule and late to go to a break, I was more likely to have an accident.

One morning at 13 WHAM, it was me and Jesse, who was fairly new in the production department, working studio camera during the morning news. Jesse had been there a few weeks and we'd worked together a handful of times. Seemed like a nice guy, a little younger than me. I was on camera one, he was running cameras two and three.

When we went to break, I ducked out to use the small bathroom that was just outside sub-control. I closed the door, locked it, pulled down my pants, sat down on the toilet, and let loose. My bowels had basically been trained at this point to know that when there was an opportunity to go, they should just fire away and get it over with.

I finished, stood up, wiped, and was washing my hands when something happened. I felt a "second wave" coming on. This was not something that had ever happened. I just stood there for a moment, frozen. I knew I didn't have time to go again. If I sat back down on the toilet now, I was not going to be back in the studio when we came back from break. But I could also tell that I really, really needed to get more out, and I needed to get it out now.

For a second, I contemplated pulling up my pants, going back to the studio, and just shitting my pants. That's right, I was standing next to a toilet and weighing the option of deliberately shitting myself. But the thing was, I felt like a *lot* more needed to come out. This was not going to be pretty.

I pulled down my pants and sat back down on the toilet. More came out. There was a sharp pain in the middle of my abdomen. It felt like a giant hand was squeezing my guts like a stress ball. I doubled over, feeling like I had gotten the wind knocked out of me.

I still had my headset on, so I could hear what was going on in sub-control and in the studio. I heard the director calling out "thirty," meaning we had thirty seconds left in the break... then "ten," and then "Check your shot, one," meaning the camera operator on camera one—which was me—needed to adjust the camera shot to get a close-up on the anchor.

I was still on the bowl and not even close to being done. Should I respond on the headset and say I wasn't going to make it back? How would I explain where I was and why? There were other people listening... the AD, the teleprompter operator, the audio engineer, the pit crew... I couldn't possibly chime in and say, "I'm in the bathroom." I just had to hope that Jesse would see I wasn't there and go adjust my camera for me. The new guy. Who had two other cameras to run. I had to hope he would run all three.

"We're out to two," the director said, meaning we were back on the air and taking camera two's shot. "Check your shot, one," she said again. I was still shitting. "One, check your shot!" she said, sounding frustrated now.

The anchors were talking. The director was able to use the two-shot of both of them from camera two and a close-up from camera three, but she couldn't cut to a close-up with camera one because it was not framed correctly and I was not there to fix it. And she kept calling, over and over, "One, check your shot!"

I was waiting for Jesse to pipe in on the headset and say, "Russ isn't here." He didn't.

After what felt like forever, Jesse must have run over to camera one, because I finally heard the director say, "Taking one," which meant she was taking the shot on camera one and putting it on the air. She sounded very annoyed.

When I finally finished in the bathroom, washed my hands, and got back into the studio, I didn't even look at anyone. Part of me wanted to go over to Jesse and say, "Hey, I'm sorry I wasn't in here when we came back from break. Thanks for covering for me. That won't happen again."

But I didn't. I couldn't even make eye contact with him. I didn't say anything to the guy. He was probably wondering what happened, where I was, and if this was something that always happened. Was it normal to be left alone in the studio to run all three cameras sometimes? He had to be wondering. I wish I would have said something, but I didn't. I just pretended that it didn't happen.

One day, I was working up in sub-control filling in as director of the twelve p.m. newscast. We were in a commercial break. A longtime member of the production crew had been helping train me on the director role after the initial training I'd had on the night shift.

"Hey, you know something I saw the other day that I thought was really gross and upsetting?" he said. He was talking not just to me but to everyone up in sub, which included the audio engineer, the producer, and the AD.

"What?" someone asked.

"I saw somebody wear one of the headsets from the studio into the bathroom," he said.

My heart stopped. The color drained from my face and everything in my body turned to stone.

"Who the hell did that?" the audio engineer exclaimed.

He hesitated for a second. "I'm not going to say who it was," he said. "I just thought that was a gross thing to do. We all have to wear those headsets. I don't want to use a headset that somebody else just wore into the bathroom."

I had not thought about that at all. When I ran into the bathroom with my headset on so I could still hear sub-control, that was a headset that someone else was going to be wearing later. It had been the farthest thing from my mind when I was going into survival mode each morning, just trying to make it through my shift.

I was mortified but also extremely grateful to the guy for not calling me out by name in front of everyone. He *had* to be talking about me. He could have completely thrown me under the bus and told everyone that I was the one who had been doing that. I would have immediately died. As it was, I felt like I wanted to crawl under the console and hide. But no one else knew he was talking about me, and he was being kind enough not to completely blow up my spot.

Going forward, any time I needed to dash to the bathroom, I took my headset off and set it on a table near the studio door. Taking the headset off and putting it back on took precious seconds off of my turnaround time. It also meant I could not hear sub-control. I would now have to rely solely on my knowledge of how long each break was and keep a close eye on my watch.

As if things weren't complicated enough already.

More than anything else, I just wanted some answers as to why I wasn't getting any better. My colonoscopy with Dr. Shreck was coming up soon. In September 2008, I sent the following email to Dr. Bill:

Hi Dr. Bill,

I just wanted to give you a quick update. I go for my colonoscopy on Monday, and I have a follow-up appointment with Dr. Shreck the following week. I have officially made the switch over to his care.

Also, I got in touch with someone from Strong about a Crohn's research study they are doing for a drug called Orencia... it is currently used for arthritis but they are finding potential with it for Crohn's. They are going to put me through the screening process to see if I qualify for the study, but the lady I talked to sounded optimistic and seems to want to try hard to get me into it.

I will keep you posted on how it turns out!

To tell you the truth, I don't have a clear memory of talking to anyone about that Orencia research study. So, obviously, nothing ever came of it. I don't remember for sure why. I think maybe you had to try and fail at Remicade first, which I had never done, or else I could not be on some of the medications I was already on to take part in the study, and I was too scared to stop taking those.

I went in for my third colonoscopy. I won't regale you with the details of the prep, as I think we have covered that pretty diligently over the course of colonoscopies one and two. The only thing I will say is that I did start the prep process much earlier than the instructions said to this time, in an effort to get ahead of the game and get it over with. The strategy paid off, and I was actually able to get some sleep that night.

This colonoscopy was different from the first two in that I woke up near the end of this one instead of being blissfully unconscious for the entire affair. I remember waking up on the table and feeling something poking around inside my guts. It didn't hurt, but it was uncomfortable. I didn't have my glasses on, so I couldn't see clearly, but I could tell that there were a few people in the room with me.

Dr. Shreck was sitting in a chair a few feet away. He was not the one conducting the exam. He was talking someone else through doing it, possibly a student or assistant who actually had the scope up my ass. I was conscious but dazed. I was not able to speak. I made a grunting, groaning noise. I was too sedated to talk but awake enough to be aware of what was going on and make sounds. I just wanted them to know that I was awake and feeling this. One of the nurses brought to Dr. Shreck's attention that I was awake.

"It's all right, we are almost finished," Dr. Shreck said. He resumed directing the assistant on what to do.

Like I said, it didn't hurt, but it was uncomfortable as hell. I could feel that there was something snaking around in my intestines, and I didn't like it. I moaned a couple more times to express my displeasure with the situation. I could see a monitor a few feet away from me showing what the scope was seeing. I tried to focus on that, because I figured that was at least a unique experience, to see your guts in real time. However, without my glasses on, I am pretty much Mr. Magoo, so all I really saw were some gray blobs.

I also remember thinking, *I don't even want pancakes after this colonoscopy. I just want to go home and go back to bed.*

Chapter Twenty-One

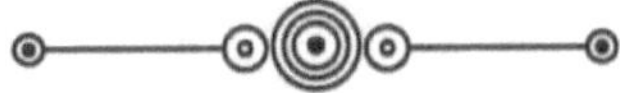

As summer turned to fall and the leaves began to change to their crisp autumn hues, a very special day was fast approaching: the date we had set for our wedding. That's right, lest you forget, dear reader, throughout all of these colonoscopies, diets, blood tests, and me working multiple jobs, my darling Amanda and I were planning a wedding this whole time!

We would be getting married at the Holy Cross Lutheran Church in Middleport, New York, where Amanda grew up. Our reception would be at the Barker Fire Hall. We were very lucky to have a lot of help and support from our family and friends.

Amanda's Aunt Sharon was the food director of a nursing home, and she was calling in some favors and taking care of all of the food for the reception and the wedding cake for us. Amanda's best friend, Amber, and her family, who are all tremendously musically talented, were going to do the music for the service. A woman I had worked with at Sam's Club had gone into the floral business and was giving us a great deal on our wedding flowers.

My cousin, who was an ordained minister, was going to give the sermon at our ceremony. We felt honored to have so many people who loved and cared about us wanting to help make our day perfect.

About two weeks before the wedding, my dad took me and a bunch of my friends out to dinner at a restaurant called The Distillery for my bachelor party. It was me, my dad, my "funcle" Al, ("funcle" means Fake Uncle; he is one of my dad's best friends and has been like an uncle to me since I was a kid), my brother, and a group of my friends. My dad was worried that the restaurant might not have anything that I could eat. He emailed me a couple of days before.

Hey Bud,

Looking forward to Sat. I would like to bring something with me that you think you may be able to eat. Please try to think of something, anything, and I'll bring it there. I could pick up a sub, or make something, or buy some pretzel-rods.

Give me a call Fri. eve, or Sat. and let me know. I'd be happy to do it.

Love,

Dad

I called him to talk about it. He said he didn't care if the restaurant had a problem with him bringing in outside food, that he would explain the situation. I told him thanks for thinking about that, but I would find something on the menu that I could order, even if I had to ask for them to make it very plain. As much as going out to eat always made me nervous, I so desperately wanted to try to feel "normal" and be able to enjoy this time leading up to the wedding as much as I possibly could.

I ended up ordering a plain hamburger and a plain baked potato. Being out to eat with family and friends filled my heart with so much happiness that day. Laughing, joking, telling old stories. For a little slice of an afternoon, I was normal.

As we were planning what songs we wanted for the wedding reception, Amanda and I picked out the songs that she would dance to with her dad and that I would dance to with my mom. For hers, she appropriately picked the song "Amanda" by Waylon Jennings. I had a harder time finding one for me and my mom. I scoured Google. One list I came upon included a song I was not familiar with—"Blessed" by Elton John. I looked it up on YouTube and listened to it. The mellow tune and loving lyrics from the point of view of a parent singing to their future child captured my heart. I sent the link to my mom and asked her what she thought of it.

This was her reply:

> *It's very pretty. Truthfully the lyrics make me a little sad, feeling we came up short in the "blessing" you department, especially when it comes to the health genes! But I guess that's part of being a parent, always wishing you could have done better for your kids. And, these dance songs are supposed to bring a tear to the eye, eh? As I said, it is very pretty. It's good with me if it's good with you.*

I felt bad that she felt that way. The fact that I had Crohn's was in no way my parents' fault! And there are all sorts of ways to be blessed. I had so many people in my life who cared about and supported me. And I had found one in particular who wanted to spend the rest of her life with me. I was indeed blessed.

It felt like the wedding preparations were taking place in a separate universe from my work life. I was very quiet at the news station, to the point that my coworkers would sometimes joke about it. Telling me to "keep it down" was a running gag, and as my wedding day approached, one of my colleagues made a remark about how the "problem" with that upcoming event was "Russ is going to have to talk."

I did not want that to be everyone's impression of me, but it was understandable. No one knew what was really going on. I was spent, running on fumes, just trying to get through my shift without collapsing from lack of sleep and horrible health. I was at every moment focused on how to get through the next block of my shift without shitting my pants.

To be very clear, I am *not* saying that I felt like anyone was being mean or picking on me. I was a good sport, and I truly have no hard feelings about it. It only bothered me in the sense that the real reason I was so quiet was that I was in physical and emotional pain every day, and having a spotlight put on it made me uncomfortable. Unfortunately, my inclination to keep to myself only drew more attention, having the exact opposite effect of what I was trying to achieve.

The original plan for the night before the wedding was going to be that Amanda was staying at her mom's house, and I was going to stay at my parents' house. I know it really meant a lot to my mom that her son was going to be at home with the family on the night before the big day. It had been her suggestion in the first place.

My Aunt Sue, Uncle Jerry, and cousin JD were coming into town for the wedding, and they were going to be staying at my parents' house as well. As the big day got closer and closer, I started to get nervous thinking about the bathroom situation. There would be eight people in the house, and only two and a half bathrooms. My Crohn's symptoms were always the worst in the morning, when everyone would need to be showering and getting ready for the wedding. I couldn't count on having free and clear access to a bathroom every time I needed it, for as long as I needed it. Just the thought of it was stressing me out. Having butterflies on the morning of your wedding was supposed to be in anticipation of saying "I do," not anxiety over whether or not the bathroom is going to be free.

Reluctantly, I told my mom I was going to spend that night in the apartment by myself instead of coming home. When I explained it, she said it would be disappointing not to have me there but that she understood.

I spent the evening alone in the apartment that I usually shared with Amanda. The next time we were both in that apartment together, we would be husband and wife.

I didn't feel nervous that night. Not really. The solitude was comforting. I slept like a baby.

Our wedding day was an absolutely gorgeous fall day, and unseasonably warm. The leaves were striking shades of red and yellow and orange, the way you would paint a picture of what autumn looks like. I rode to the church with my parents, my Great-Aunt Marian, and one of my groomsmen, Mark, my good friend since high school.

All morning, everyone kept asking me, "Are you nervous?" And quite honestly, the answer was no, I was not nervous. At least, I was not nervous about marrying Amanda. Of course the thought was, as always, in the back of my mind, *I hope I don't shit my pants.* Usually when you hear about guys getting cold feet before the wedding, it's not them wondering whether or not they are going to literally soil their tux.

I needed to be as prepared as possible. I took some Imodium about an hour or so before the wedding to slow things down in there. That meant I would be paying for it later when things got moving again and I was going to have some cramps, but it should buy me the better part of the day without having to go to the bathroom. The last thing I needed was to be in the middle of our vows and have to ask Amanda to hold that thought. I also wore two pairs of underwear, with a whole bunch of toilet paper lining the inside, to act as a sort of makeshift diaper in case things went south. When my groomsmen and I were downstairs in the church basement changing into our tuxes, I tried to change my pants as quickly as possible so no one would notice my unusual underwear modifications.

Before long, it was time for us to file in upstairs. There I was, standing at the front of the sanctuary, looking out over the faces of all of the guests. Friends that I had known since high school. Family members, some of whom I had not seen in years. Amanda's relatives, some of whom I knew very well while others were total strangers to me. All sitting there, watching and waiting, gathering in this one place on this one specific day to watch me and Amanda get married.

Okay, yeah, now I was starting to get nervous. Stage-fright, butterflies nervous. Everyone was looking at me. I was in the spotlight on display. Vulnerable. I was not comfortable being the center of attention. I had gotten so used to just blending in, staying in the background, being inconspicuous. This was the polar opposite.

The bridesmaids and groomsmen entered in pairs. My brother, Josh, was my best man. Amanda's sister, Anne, was her maid of honor. Their entrances were all beautifully accompanied by music from Amber's family. It was all playing out in front of me like a movie while I was very much in my own head. I had that jittery kind of nervous feeling, like when you're going up the first huge hill of a roller-coaster.

Until Amanda walked in. As soon as I saw her in her dress for the first time, I felt at ease. Her dress, with its majestically flowing train, was absolutely gorgeous, and it looked perfect on her. Her smile was as bright and white as her dress. As Amanda's father walked her down the aisle, my nervousness dissipated like parting clouds revealing a ray of sunshine. There she was—my partner, my best friend, my bride. She and I were in this together, just like we were in everything together. I had felt nervous because I had been up there all alone. I wasn't alone anymore. And I never would be again.

Amanda's dad placed her hand on my arm. We took the final steps toward the altar together. We looked at each other and smiled. There was such a feeling of "we made it." We made it to this day, to this place, to this moment.

The service was such a special and personal celebration of our love and of the people in our lives. Amber sang "The Wedding Song" as we lit our unity candle. Amanda's brother and his wife read the Bible verses. My cousin delivered a sermon that brought the house down, quoting not only the immortal words of scripture, "Love never fails," but the sage wisdom of Peter Parker's Uncle Ben, "With great power comes great responsibility."

The moment that struck me the hardest and has continued to stay with me ever since was when we were saying our vows. I could not help but be overcome by the words "in sickness and in health." Amanda had already paid more than her fair share of dues in that category. She had been by my side faithfully through so much sickness. I only hoped that I could get healthy soon so we could start enjoying some truly good times, not just enduring bad ones together.

Amanda and I walked into our reception at the Barker Fire Hall to a thunderous standing ovation as "Some Fantastic" by Barenaked Ladies played. With Amanda on my arm, I felt safe being the center of attention. This day wasn't about me, it was about us. And "us" was something I was glad to be celebrating.

The food at the reception was legendary, and our guests still talk about it to this day. Aunt Sharon and her crew prepared a veritable Thanksgiving feast, served buffet style. Turkey, stuffing, mashed potatoes, cranberry sauce, corn, enough to feed an army. Everyone was raving about how good the food was. I couldn't eat any of it, of course, but Aunt Sharon took care of that too—she discreetly gave me my own special plate of well-done roast beef, a plain baked potato, and very soft boiled carrots. These were all things I felt safe eating. I didn't feel bad that I couldn't enjoy the feast our guests were having. I was used to that by now. I was just glad I had something I could eat, and that our loved ones were having a great time.

The cake was an unbelievable multi-layer work of art that looked like a snapshot of a fairy tale. There were glass figurines of a man and woman dancing in the middle, and stairs leading to even more layers of cake above them, as if they were in the middle of a kind of confectionary castle. In front of the cake, a glass horse-drawn chariot awaited the couple when they finished their dance, and red and brown leaves were strewn about the carriage, mirroring the real-life fall scenery outside. Amanda and I cut the cake and delicately fed each other a small forkful. That solitary bite would be all that I ate of the cake. Sugary sweets were just one more thing that tended to send my stomach into spasms. That single bite tasted like heaven. We didn't smash cake into each other's faces; instead, we playfully pasted a dollop of frosting onto one another's noses. It was cute. Amanda was always so gentle and careful with me. It was beyond endearing.

The lights dimmed, and the DJ called us to the middle of the room for our first dance together as husband and wife. We had decided on a song that was very special to us: "When You Wish Upon a Star," as sung by Billy Joel. The soft, sweet melody began to play as I took my blushing bride in my arms. As we swayed gently back and forth to the music, I thought about the contrast between the two times we had danced to this song. The first, just the two of us in Virginia, far away from everyone else that we knew, dancing by the light of the Christmas tree. And now, celebrating our love surrounded by so many people who cared about us, starting a new chapter of our story together. The lyrics "your dreams come true" seemed like they were being sung directly to us.

Despite how hard everything else had been for me lately, this one day got to be absolutely perfect. It really was like a fairy tale.

We took a modest honeymoon at the Briars Resort on Lake Simcoe, which is north of Toronto, Canada. We got married on a Saturday and left for the resort on Tuesday. I went to work on the Monday in between. Since I didn't have any paid time off from 13 WHAM, taking time off meant a smaller paycheck, and to say that money was tight was the understatement of the year. We had briefly considered not taking a honeymoon at all in order to save money but ultimately decided that we deserved, or in fact downright needed, some quality time together as husband and wife.

Amanda and I got to the resort in the early afternoon on Tuesday. We stayed in a small private cabin in a secluded wooded area that was just a short walk from the calm and tranquil lake. The cabin was quaint, homey, and surrounded by the serenity of nature. Just up the road was a main lodge that served three meals a day, included in the price of our stay.

Breakfast was the best by far, as they had a huge buffet with every type of breakfast food you could imagine. This made it easy for me to load up on things I knew were relatively safe for me to eat, like scrambled eggs and toast. Lunch was also served buffet style, but it was harder for me to find things that I could have on my limited diet.

Dinner was not served buffet style and instead had a sit-down menu. There would be a list of a few appetizers, entrees, and desserts, and you could pick one of each as part of the all-inclusive package. The food was a little too fancy for our tastes. I could usually manage to find something on the menu that I could handle, although I'd have to leave a salad or side dish untouched.

It seems like the fancier a place is, the more likely they are to have skins in their mashed potatoes. The skin was hard for me to digest, so I would have to pick around it or just skip it altogether. One night, burnt out on the elegant cuisine of the resort, we looked at each other and were like, "Want to just go out for a burger?" We blew off the three-course meal we were entitled to, drove up the road to a bar and grill, and got hamburgers and fries.

The resort had a very nice spa on site, and one day Amanda and I went for massages. There was an incredible shower with about a dozen jets spraying you from all angles that you went in before and after your massage. It was extremely relaxing and definitely just right for the quiet, get-away-from-it-all honeymoon that we wanted.

Another luxury at the lodge was a huge indoor pool. Because there were not many people staying there—keep in mind, we were way up north, and this was October—we were able to take a few dips in the pool and have it all to ourselves. Most of the time this was awesome, but one afternoon, we were in the pool and I got that intense squeezing feeling in my lower abdomen. I knew I had to go to the bathroom ASAP. I hopped out of the pool.

"Where are you going?" Amanda asked.

"I'll be right back!" I called, sprint-waddling down the hallway to the restrooms. I was trying not to slip on the wet tile floor, but also hurrying my ass to the bathroom so I wouldn't have an accident.

I got to the men's room just in time. Well, almost just in time. I pulled my swim trunks down at the last second and plopped down onto the toilet… only to find that I had gotten some excrement in my trunks. I couldn't believe it. I punched the stall wall. This was my honeymoon! Why was I having to deal with this?

After I finished going, I had to try to get the poop out of the lining of my trunks. It was impossible to get all of it out, clinging to the small wet holes in the mesh lining. Without taking them off and really washing and scrubbing them good with soap and water, I was not going to be able to get it all out. I gritted my teeth and cursed. I felt like crying. Why was this happening? I was supposed to be in the pool with my wife right now, not trying to get shit out of my shorts.

Eventually I just pulled the trunks back up after getting them as clean as I could, but I knew I had not gotten everything. There was more than a skid mark still in there. I knew I could not go back in the pool like that. I would be contaminating the pool with fecal matter and creating a potential health hazard. I was going to have to tell my new bride, "Hey, honey, I can't get back in the water. I just shit my swimming trunks."

When I got back to the pool, Amanda had already gotten out and was sitting on a chair, looking upset. "Well, are you ready to go?" she asked.

"Oh... do you not want to get back in the pool?" I asked hesitantly.

"No. I got out, because I didn't want to be in there by myself," she said sadly. "And now I'm dry, so I don't really want to get back in. Let's just go back to the cabin."

"Oh. Okay. If you're sure," I said.

I had dodged a bullet... kind of. I didn't have to tell Amanda what had happened. But I had also ruined our pool time and made Amanda sad. I couldn't help but think back to what Amanda had said at that support group meeting. That sometimes she felt like she had Crohn's too. My limitations became her limitations.

And now they would be her limitations until death do us part.

Chapter Twenty-Two

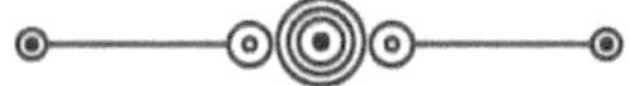

Back to the real world after our getaway. In October 2008, I was willing to give anything a shot, and I started seeing a hypnotherapist. Dr. Yeardley was a psychologist who, among other services, offered hypnosis as a way to treat eating disorders, anxiety, and digestive issues, including Crohn's disease. Nothing else had worked so far, so I figured I might as well give this a try.

The drive to Dr. Yeardley's office was about twenty minutes from the apartment. I was always willing to try something new if I thought there was even a chance that it could help me, but it was always very draining. Just the commitment of the time and energy to drive out somewhere, have the appointment, and drive back, coupled with the anxiety I would have about being somewhere unfamiliar, not knowing what the bathroom situation would be, was physically and mentally exhausting.

Dr. Yeardley's office was small and had stuff all over the place. It looked like she was perpetually in the middle of spring cleaning and hadn't figured out where anything was going to go.

I sat down in a recliner at the far end of the office, and Dr. Yeardley sat down in a rocking chair a few feet away. We went over my history, what I had tried so far to treat my Crohn's. I gave her the whole laundry list. By now I could recite it all off the top of my head. She felt that she could help me and asked my permission to hypnotize me. I said sure.

Dr. Yeardley told me to lean back in the chair and get into a comfortable position, one that I would be okay to stay still in for a while without needing to move around too much. She said I could recline back in the chair and put my feet up if I wanted to. I did so. She had me look up at a spot on the ceiling. Because I was looking upward, it was like I was letting my eyes roll back in my head.

"Just concentrate on that spot and listen to my words," she said. "And at the same time, I want you to start to relax your body."

She told me that she was going to count from one to three, and that as she did so, a heavy feeling would start to come into my eyelids. They would become heavier and heavier until my eyelids would finally sink down and I would close my eyes automatically.

"One… relax your body. Allow it to become heavy and limp. And as you do, your eyelids also begin to feel heavier and heavier. And soon they will start pushing down, more and more. Two… now take a deep breath, a very deep breath… and exhale very slowly… your eyelids are becoming heavier, feel the heaviness in your eyelids, as if they are weighted down…"

By the time she got to three, my eyes were shut and I was feeling copacetic.

Once my eyes were closed, Dr. Yeardley told me she wanted me to picture myself standing at the top of a very large marble staircase, covered by a rich, velvety carpet. She took her time painting the picture of what this staircase looked like, what the carpet felt like, really encouraged me to picture this in my mind's eye in as much detail as I could. She wanted me to picture myself walking down the steps, that she was going to talk me through taking each step one by one, and that as I descended the staircase, I was going to be going deeper and deeper into a hypnotic state.

"One. Take the first step down. Feel the wonderful softness of the carpet under your feet as you stand there on the first step below. As I continue to count, you'll go down one step further with each number. At the same time, going deeper and deeper into the hypnotic state, effortlessly and automatically, deeper and deeper with each number. The color of the carpet on the steps in front of you becomes deeper and deeper with each step down. A deeper and more restful color with each step you take. Two. Now you take another step down…"

As she kept talking, something strange happened. Her voice started to sound farther and farther away. It was like there was a tunnel separating us, and she was slipping down the tunnel. Or maybe like someone was very gradually turning down the volume on a radio. I was feeling very relaxed, and the world just seemed to be fading away around me.

The next thing I knew, Dr. Yeardley was saying, "Three… you're almost about to open your eyes. Two… you're very close to opening your eyes. And one… you open your eyes fully and are wide awake, relaxed and comfortable, inside and out."

And as I opened my eyes and looked around the room, I realized a decent chunk of time had passed between when her voice was starting to get far away in the tunnel and just now. And I had not been aware of that time passing.

"How do you feel?" she asked.

"Um… that… was very weird," I said.

"How so?" she asked cheerfully.

"I remember you talking me through walking down the steps," I said, "and I remember the first couple of steps on the staircase… and then your voice started to sound really far away, and then I don't remember anything else until you brought me out of it just now."

Dr. Yeardley was smiling. "But you heard it," she assured me. "Your mind heard it. The mind is an amazing thing. It heard everything I said, and your mind will still process it, even if you were not consciously aware of it."

For a moment, I had an embarrassing thought. "Could I have fallen asleep?"

Dr. Yeardley considered the question for a moment. "No," she said. "No, I don't think so, Russ. I was watching your face, and I would have known if you were asleep. Being asleep looks different than being hypnotized."

I figured it also would have been quite a coincidence if I had fallen asleep and then just happened to wake up as Dr. Yeardley was doing the last few numbers of her countdown to bring me back out of it. I was amazed. I had not really known what to expect, but I sure didn't expect to go into some kind of trance! And I really did feel relaxed and refreshed.

Before I left, we scheduled my next appointment for two weeks out. Dr. Yeardley said that the sessions needed to be spaced out regularly to be effective, and two weeks was the recommended interval. I should plan on coming every other week for a total of seven sessions.

It was a Wednesday. I went and visited my parents in the afternoon like I usually did on Wednesdays. I was excited to tell them about my experience with hypnosis. They were amazed when I told them about how I didn't remember any of the session, how I had "gone under" so much that I had no idea what was said. My dad joked that next time someone snapped their fingers, I was going to start clucking like a chicken.

The best part? I wasn't making my usual urgent sprints to the bathroom that afternoon. I had to go a few times, but that extreme urgency was not there, and that overall sense of unease and being on edge was not there either. I felt more relaxed, and my parents even commented that I seemed more comfortable. Were we really onto something here?

Two weeks later, I was happy to go back. Would I go into a trance again? What would it feel like if I was expecting it this time? Would I be able to tell when I was going under? Mostly, I was looking forward to feeling relaxed and refreshed like I did after my first session.

Except that's not what happened.

I leaned back in the chair just like the first time. I listened to Dr. Yeardley telling me again that I was going to feel more and more relaxed. That my eyelids were going to start to feel heavy, that I could close them when I felt like I couldn't keep them open anymore. I waited for that moment to come. But it didn't. And as Dr. Yeardley continued talking, eventually I was past the point in the monologue where I should have my eyes closed, so I just went ahead and shut them. I didn't feel like I physically had to, like before. I felt like I was "falling behind," so I just did it.

As she continued talking, soothingly telling me that I was becoming more and more relaxed and that I was going deeper into my own mind, I kept waiting for something to happen. I was looking for that moment of falling into the trance, of the tunnel and the quieting radio. Instead, I actually felt more alert, like I was hyper-aware of everything. I felt fidgety instead of relaxed. I was on edge, waiting for "it" to happen. Waiting for that moment of going under. It never came.

This time, I got to hear Dr. Yeardley's entire narrative. After walking down the twenty steps of the marble staircase, you walk outside to a grassy meadow. Then, after walking through the meadow, you come to a lake where a boat is tied up on a dock. Then you get in the boat and sail to a small, peaceful island. On the island, you feel completely at peace and in control of your body and your bowels. You will take that feeling back with you and keep it after the session is over. You get back in the boat, sail back, go back across the meadow, go back up the stairs and three, two, one, your eyes open.

Dr. Yeardley could tell I was disappointed. I wasn't trying to hide the frown on my face.

"How do you feel?' she asked, more hesitant this time.

"It didn't work like last time."

"What do you mean by that?" she asked.

"I never 'went under' this time. I was aware of everything. I heard every word you were saying."

"That's okay," Dr. Yeardley said. "Just because you didn't go into a deep trance like you did last time, doesn't mean that it didn't work. You don't need to go all the way under to feel the benefits of the hypnosis."

We scheduled my next appointment for two weeks out.

Had I ruined the session by not letting myself relax? I had been so hyper-aware of everything because I was anticipating that moment of going under. I wanted to feel it happening again, and I psyched myself out. And then, even as the whole session was going on, I was not relaxed and was not really getting into it because I was stressing out that I was not doing it right, telling myself that I had messed it up, worrying that it was not working. As happy and relaxed as I had been after the first session, I was just as bummed leaving this one.

My next session two weeks later was pretty much the same. I was so eager to feel that moment of "going under" again that I never got there. Again, I spent the whole session kicking myself because I wasn't relaxing enough, which in turn made it impossible to relax. Now I started to wonder again if maybe I had just fallen asleep during that first session after all.

As 2008 was nearing its end, something quite amazing happened. I had reached my out-of-pocket maximum for my insurance policy for that year. This meant that I had spent so much money on prescriptions, doctor appointments, lab tests, etc. that everything for the rest of the year would be covered 100% by insurance. My prescription refills, my copays, everything would be at absolutely no charge to me until the end of the year. It was a miracle, although it was an expensive miracle. The out-of-pocket maximum for my policy was $5,000. I had spent five grand on medical expenses in less than a year.

As I was scheduling an appointment with Dr. Yeardley in early December, I mentioned this to her. She said we could go ahead and fit my remaining appointments in before the end of the year. So we scheduled four appointments in December. While I was appreciative of the fact that I was going to get four sessions at no cost to me, it did strike me as a little odd that in our first session she'd said spacing the sessions out every two weeks would be the most effective frequency, and now I was going to be getting them only a week apart. I didn't question it, but it did make me wonder what we were really doing here.

My remaining sessions continued on the same way all the others had after that first one. I never achieved that full state of being in a trance like I did in the first session again. At my very last session, Dr. Yeardley gave me a CD that she had recorded just for me with the meditation on it, so I could listen to it whenever I needed to. I was glad that she did that, but also by this time kind of feeling like maybe this was just not going to do the trick for me at all. Appropriately, every time I tried listening to the CD at home, I fell asleep.

Meanwhile, my incontinence at work was getting really bad. Even with how often I was running to the bathroom, there were still times that I just could not make it. I was too far away or didn't have enough time. Continuing with what I had started on my wedding day, I was wearing two pairs of underwear every day now, with toilet paper crammed into them to try to absorb anything that came out and make for easier clean-up.

One day I was back in the editing bay, and I knew I was about to have an accident. I could tell that even if I absolutely sprinted from the edit bay to the bathroom (which I was not about to do) I was not going to make it in time. I stood up, took a few deep breaths, and just tried to stay as calm as I could as I soiled myself.

Except this time, instead of only defecating in my pants, the contraction in my abdomen was so intense that I also peed myself. Despite what Billy Madison would have us believe, peeing your pants is not cool.

Fortunately, the fact that I was wearing two pairs of underwear with a layer of toilet paper lining them, and also wearing dark jeans, meant that you could not tell that I had wet my pants. I slowly sauntered to the bathroom for my usual clean-up ritual, but this was really concerning. The only other time I had urinated during an accident was that time I shit the bed when all of our friends were leaving for that wine tour. Was this going to keep happening? Now I not only had to worry about stuff coming out the back end, but the front end was fair game too? This was getting more complicated.

I decided my makeshift diapers were not going to cut it. It was time for me to get some real ones.

After work, I stopped by Walmart and bought a pack of Depends adult diapers.

I was mortified to be buying them. I was worried about what the cashier would think. I decided that I was not buying them for myself. I was buying them for my grandfather. Grandpa asked me to buy him some adult diapers, can you believe it?

Not that I would tell the cashier this. It was just a narrative I was building in my head. In these few minutes that I was waiting in line and purchasing these diapers, I was in a fictitious world where I was not the one who needed them. I was doing my grandpa a favor and getting them for him. I had to believe that lie, myself, in my mind, as I went through the checkout just to be able to go through with it. Never mind the fact that one of my grandfathers was deceased and the other one lived in Atlanta, and as far as I knew, neither of them wore diapers at any point. I had to mentally become someone else to make that purchase.

I developed a new routine. I had a light black-and-gray jacket that I wore to 13 WHAM every day. The lights that the anchors were under in the studio got pretty hot, so the temperature in the studio itself was kept quite cold. Wearing the jacket all the time did not seem conspicuous. The jacket had big zip-up pockets. In each pocket, I stashed an extra diaper and a plastic grocery bag. That way, if I had an accident, the next time I was able to sneak into the bathroom, I was able to change the diaper for a new one, put the soiled one in a plastic bag, tie it shut, and bury it at the bottom of the garbage under some paper towels.

I did not tell Amanda that I was doing this. I was so embarrassed about it, I just didn't know how to tell her. I didn't want her to know I was having accidents at work almost every day now. It just felt so gross, and I was honestly ashamed by it.

Money was tight going into the holiday season of 2008. After spending $5,000 on medical expenses over the course of the year, I badly needed to replenish my bank account, and I wanted to have some money to buy Christmas presents. We were also starting to talk about moving out of the apartment and had been looking at houses here and there.

In an effort to bank some extra hours, I asked the manager of the business office at Sam's Club if I could pick up some extra shifts during the week instead of just working there on the weekend. I also let the front-end managers know I'd be willing to work cashier some afternoons/evenings if they needed me to.

This resulted in some days in November and December where I was working 3:30 a.m. to 12:30 p.m. at 13 WHAM, and then 2:00 p.m. to 7:00 p.m. at Sam's Club. There was even a Saturday that I picked up an extra shift at 13 WHAM and ended up working 7:00 a.m. to 2:30 p.m. at Sam's Club and 3:00 p.m. to midnight at 13 WHAM.

It was insane. A healthy person would be exhausted by that kind of schedule, and I was about as far from healthy as you could get. But in my mind, it was worth it as a temporary measure to be able to sack some money away. It made Christmas something I was looking forward to even more, because I was going to stop pulling double duty after that and go back to "just" working one job a day, seven days a week!

In mid-December, I had another appointment with Dr. Shreck. I had lost five pounds since my last visit. I knew why I was losing weight: I had become afraid to eat. Any food going in had to come out, right? Eating less would mean less bowel movements, wouldn't it? If I wanted to minimize how much time I was spending on the toilet, I should minimize the amount of food I was eating. I don't know if I actually sat down and thought through it in quite those terms or if it was just becoming an unconscious habit, but that negative association with eating was becoming forged in my brain either way.

Dr. Shreck was advising me to try tapering off the prednisone again, decreasing it by 1 mg every two weeks, and he had me discontinue the 6-MP that Dr. Griswold had started me on. Dr. Shreck also prescribed me another new medication, called Bentyl, also known as dicyclomine. It was an anti-spasmodic. Because I had met my out-of-pocket maximum, the appointment and prescription were at no cost to me.

I started taking the Bentyl in late December. I was not optimistic. We'd tried so many things, and I got my hopes up each time with every new addition only to have them dashed when it didn't work. I was starting to feel less hopeful and more skeptical with each new treatment we tried.

So imagine my surprise when, after taking Bentyl only a couple of times, I started to feel relief. That incessant urge that always had me sprinting for the toilet was just not there. That always-on-edge, never-quite-comfortable tightness in my lower abdomen subsided. My bowels actually felt calm. I couldn't believe it. I was able to go hours, sometimes even the better part of a day, without needing to run to the restroom. Had we finally hit on something that worked?

I was prescribed this medication to be taken every six hours as needed. At first I was taking it when I got up in the morning, another dose around midday, and one more in the evening, and it was working great.

After a couple of weeks of taking it, I noticed that it was starting to wear off a little sooner. When it would be almost time for the next dose, my stomach would start to cramp up, and I'd start to feel that uncomfortable tension again. I'd find myself running to the bathroom once or twice as it got really close to being time for the next dose. No big deal, I thought. Most of my day still brought me a lot of relief. Maybe I could start taking the doses a little closer together, as long as I was still keeping it within that six-hour margin.

The problem was, this window kept getting smaller and smaller. The interlude between spikes in my symptoms was growing shorter every day, and the time I spent with that great sense of relief was dwindling.

We spent New Year's Eve at Amanda's mom's house. The "rebound effect" of the Bentyl, as I was calling it, had reached unfathomable levels. I was now only getting an hour or two of relief from my symptoms after a dose, and when the symptoms came back, they were more intense than ever. It was like those periods of relief were just saving up the agony, and then I'd get it all back compounded with interest.

I spent most of that New Year's Eve in the bathroom, because when the Bentyl wore off, I was hit with painful diarrhea and the sensation that my colon was being crushed in a vise. Once it started, it was constant. I could not leave the bathroom. Amanda had to ask everyone else if they could stay out of the main bathroom so that I could use it as much as I needed, and if they could use the one off the master bedroom instead. It was pure misery, made worse by the fact that I was not at home and was embarrassingly out of commission in front of everyone. Worst of all, I'd gotten my hopes up higher than ever when the Bentyl had been working so well.

I stopped taking the Bentyl.

Happy fucking New Year.

Chapter Twenty-Three

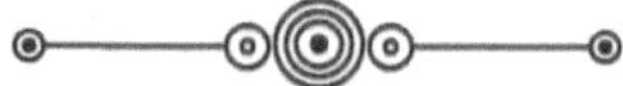

As 2009 kicked off, we made plans with Amanda's sister, Anne, and her boyfriend to go to a Buffalo Sabres hockey game to celebrate the girls' birthdays, which are only a day apart. We grabbed tickets for the Sabres vs. New York Rangers game at HSBC Arena in Buffalo. I was so tired from working constantly that I asked Amanda if she would mind driving. She said no problem. I dozed off a few times on the hour or so drive from Rochester to Buffalo.

I woke up with a start to the all-too-familiar tense, tight feeling in the pit of my stomach. "Uggh," I groaned. "Honey, I need to go to the bathroom. Can we stop somewhere?"

We were in downtown Buffalo but not quite to the arena.

"Umm," Amanda said. "Yes, let me see what's around…"

We were in a busy area with a lot of traffic and not a lot of places to stop. There were no gas stations or convenience stores in sight, just office buildings and parking garages. Nowhere that looked suitable for a quick pop-in to use the restroom.

"I don't think we are very far from the arena," Amanda said. "Do you think you can make it?"

"No," I said, shifting uncomfortably in my seat. Even if we had been pulling into the damn arena, I didn't think I could make it. The time it would take to find a parking place, walk into the building, and find the bathroom would have been too much to ask. "Can we find a restaurant or something?"

"Okay, okay, let me see what I can do," Amanda said. She was looking down side streets, trying to figure out where we could turn off. "I think there might be some down this way…" She made a quick right turn. We drove past more businesses, and even a couple of bars and diners, but the streets were so packed with people heading to the game that there was nowhere to park. I closed my eyes as the tightness in my gut became worse.

"I don't think I'm going to make it," I whimpered.

"Hold on, I see a diner up ahead. Just hang on, Russ, we can make it."

Amanda pulled into the parking lot of a mom-and-pop-style family diner and grabbed a spot right in front. And just as she did so, I lost control of my bowels and shit my pants.

"Okay, we're here," Amanda said, looking at me quizzically because I was still just sitting there. "Go ahead."

My face was screwed up in an expression of pain and shame.

"It's too late," I said. "I didn't make it."

"Oh." She frowned. "I… aw. I'm sorry. I got here as fast as I could…"

"It's not your fault."

"Do you… want to go in, and clean up…?"

"No," I said. "I don't want to go into this random restaurant and use their bathroom and clean up. Just… just get us to the arena. I'll clean up there."

"Are you sure?" Amanda said. "I mean, I know we're close, but…"

"I'm sure. I don't want to shuffle into the restaurant past whoever is seating people and change my underwear and then just come back out. I just don't want to. Just get us to the arena. Please." I was frustrated but not at Amanda. I hoped she didn't think I was snapping at her, even though I kind of was. I was mad at my life.

When we arrived at the arena, I made my way to a bathroom, shit some more into the toilet this time, and changed my diaper to a spare one that I had in my jacket pocket. Amanda still didn't know that I wore Depends at this point. She didn't ask for the details of how I'd cleaned up, and I didn't offer them.

By the time we got to our seats, we had missed the start of the game, and the Sabres had scored a few goals already. I was so dejected. This was my wife's birthday. It was supposed to be a fun outing to celebrate. Once again, my disease had ruined something that should have been special.

On top of everything else we were dealing with at this point, Amanda and I were in the process of house hunting. Funcle Al, who I mentioned earlier, was a real estate agent. He was showing us some houses, mostly in the Greece and Henrietta areas.

One Friday evening in January, we went to look at a house and my dad came with us. I was feeling especially sick that night. I was so tired that I was walking around in a stupor, barely paying attention or looking around the place. I felt so ill that a couple of times I had to surreptitiously break off from the group and go use the bathroom. That's right, I defecated in the bathroom of the house we were looking at, and more than once.

The next day my mom sent me this email:

After seeing you last night, Dad is very worried about you, and so am I. We talked about it briefly last night, but he was so concerned he called me at work this morning to talk some more. We are both very worried about you and I have to put my two cents in.

First, you HAVE to stop working so much. You have to have at least one day off a week, and preferably two. Even a person in outstanding health cannot keep up the pace you are without affecting their health, and you are not in outstanding health to begin with. If you can't afford to buy a house without the second job, then buying a house will have to wait. Period. Your health has to come first. No house or any other material possession is worth pushing yourself the way you are.

Second, Dad and I both think you should not buy that house. Such a big decision is not something you should be making in your current condition. Pass on the house, take some time to get yourself better again, and then think about house buying. More and more houses will be put on the market as we move into spring. Right now you need to take a break from Sam's, rest, and take care of yourself!

Please forgive me butting in, but we love you and are very worried about you! When he called me at work this morning, Dad said, "I used to be worried about his health. Now I'm worried about his life!" I sincerely hope that his concern is exaggerated, but you never know. When one is talking about one's health—and life—better safe than sorry! You can't keep working seven days a week! Your health HAS to come first! Please listen to us and put the second job and the house hunting on a back burner for now and make taking care of yourself the priority!

The fact that my parents were fearing for my life at this point shook me up. I couldn't help but think back to that diagnosis from Dr. Harvey. *You will have a shorter life span.* Was I literally killing myself? At the same time, I didn't know what to do. My mom was saying I needed to take a break from work. But how would I do that? I was struggling to pay my medical bills as it was. I was stuck in a cycle of doom and didn't know how to get out of it.

Still, my parents were absolutely not wrong that my health was the worst it had been. Per that last visit with Dr. Shreck, I was once again trying to taper off of the prednisone. I got down to 5 mg per day, and then the severe symptoms of intense abdominal pain, extremely urgent bowel movements, and blood in my stool came back. That low of a dose just was not enough to keep the most extreme symptoms at bay.

I had lost another ten pounds since my previous visit the month prior; I was down to 140 now. I wasn't scheduled to see Dr. Shreck again for a few more months, but the shape I was in was so bad, it prompted me to call his office and try to get in as soon as possible. I told them what a bad state I was in. They told me to go for bloodwork as soon as I could so they could check my CRP levels, and they scheduled me an appointment to come back in and see Dr. Shreck.

Amanda drove me to the appointment. On the way there, I had something I wanted to tell her, but I wasn't sure how to bring it up. I sat in silence for a long time trying to figure out the right way to say it. It wasn't something to just easily segue into.

"You would love me no matter what, right?"

Amanda looked at me out of the side of her eye and raised an eyebrow. "Of course I would…" she said genuinely, but with concern in her voice.

"There's something I have to tell you, and it's really embarrassing," I said. I felt so awkward. I looked down at my feet.

"What is it?" she asked. "You know you can tell me anything."

I hesitated. "I… um… I don't know. There's not really an easy way to say it." I was dragging it out so much, which was only making it worse. But I felt like it needed some kind of lead-in, only there really was no way to preamble this piece of information.

Finally, after much hemming and hawing, I said it.

"I've been wearing adult diapers to work every day. And, just, pretty much all the time, in general. Because I keep having times where I can't make it to the bathroom in time. I've been wearing them for a while, but I just never really found the right time or the right way to tell you. It's a weird thing to bring up. But I'm telling you now because I'm going to bring it up at my appointment today, and I didn't want that to be the first time you heard about it."

I paused. Amanda did not look disgusted, upset, or even surprised for that matter. She gave me a gentle, comforting smile. She reached over and took my hand and gave it a small squeeze.

"Hey," she said. "I'm glad you're doing that. That must be really helpful. I know how stressful it is for you, especially when you're working at the station, to not know if you're going to be able to get to the bathroom when you need to. I bet it helps you have some peace of mind to be wearing that. Good for you."

How had I ever thought that she would react any other way? She was always so supportive of me. Always in my corner, no matter what.

At the appointment, as usual, we saw Lorraine first and filled her in on everything that had been going on. I told her about how the Bentyl had worked great at first, but the rebound effect became unbearable and that I had stopped taking it. I told her how the urgency, discomfort, and blood in the stool had gotten exponentially worse at this low dose of prednisone. She noted my weight loss, and I told her how I was afraid to eat. She referred to this as anorexia, which I had not considered it to be, but I suppose it was. I also told her that I had been wearing adult diapers to work because I was basically incontinent at this point. She gave me a very sympathetic look when I told her that. This was a woman who heard this kind of stuff all day every day, and I could tell that the state that I was in was affecting her.

Dr. Shreck came in and listened to the recap.

Dr. Shreck's response was to up my prednisone dose back to 40 mg a day. I was now going back on a dose that was just as high as I'd been on back in August 2007 when I was hospitalized for that first bad Crohn's flare-up. Was I ever going to get off of this stuff?

But Dr. Shreck would drop an even bigger bombshell on me than upping the prednisone dose.

He did not think that I had Crohn's disease.

The biopsies from my colonoscopy in September showed active proctitis of the rectum and left colon, while the right colon and terminal ilium showed no chronic inflammation or histological abnormalities. The serology markers showed a pattern more consistent with ulcerative colitis than Crohn's disease. As such, he was changing my diagnosis from Crohn's to colitis.

To me, this seemed like it should have been a huge revelation. Did this mean we had been treating it wrong the whole time? Was this a breakthrough that was going to come with a new path forward? Dr. Shreck did not really seem to think so.

"The treatment for Crohn's disease and ulcerative colitis is essentially the same," Dr. Shreck said. "We treat the inflammation and bring it down. It does not really matter much which one you have."

He said he wanted to see me again in two weeks.

The whole drive home, I thought about the fact that I, apparently, did not have Crohn's, but actually had colitis. I also thought back to the day Dr. Harvey had diagnosed me and said, "For lack of a better term, you have Crohn's disease." That phrasing had stuck in the back of my mind and was coming back to haunt me now. Had it been too close to call back then, and Dr. Harvey basically just guessed?

Dr. Shreck may have said it did not really matter, but it mattered to me. Having Crohn's disease had become part of my identity. It wasn't exactly something I was proud of, but it was a part of who I was. It was a name for my pain. It was a battle I had been fighting, something I had been trying so hard to overcome. What it actually was mattered a lot to me. Finding out that it was (possibly? probably?) colitis felt, somehow, disappointing. Especially when that revelation did not come with any kind of step forward in my treatment.

I also couldn't help but think about how Dr. Shreck had had me take the breath test that had shown I wasn't lactose intolerant, after Dr. Griswold had said that I was. Was Dr. Shreck just determined to negate the results of my previous doctors, like a judge overturning a court case? It almost felt like some kind of power trip. But how was I supposed to know what was right or wrong at this point? I was more confused than ever.

I refilled the prednisone. I had 5 mg tablets. I had been taking one a day. Now I was taking eight—four in the morning and four before bed.

As I was taking my evening dose, I grumbled about how much I hated being on it and how I wished I didn't have to go back to such a high dose of it. Amanda innocently asked why I felt that way when it was clear that it did help my symptoms get back under control.

"Because it makes me feel like shit!" I yelled, and I threw the bottle of pills at the wall. It narrowly missed hitting Amanda in the head.

I apologized immediately. The span of time between me throwing the bottle and saying I was sorry was about three seconds.

It's difficult to describe the way prednisone made me feel better and worse at the same time. When I got down to the low doses, my symptoms got dialed up to eleven. Rectal bleeding, extreme urgency, and constantly feeling like there were knives tumbling around inside my lower abdomen. When I upped the prednisone to a high dose, the bleeding would go away and that razor-sharp pain would subside, but I'd be trading that for a dark, gloomy cloud of bitterness that seemed to overtake my mind. The steroid turned me into an angry jackass who wanted to punch the world in the face.

On top of that, it's not like it even put me into full remission. It took that extreme edge off of my pain, but I was still taking a couple dozen trips to the bathroom every day, and that's not an exaggeration. It was simply trading one form of misery for another.

My next visit to Dr. Shreck was in February 2009. I had gained a few pounds back since the last time I was there. I felt better compared to the abysmal low I had been at the last time I was there, but I was still in rough shape.

So that's why it was surprising to me when Dr. Shreck told me that I was all better.

He had the results of my most recent bloodwork up on the computer screen, and calmly told me that because my CRP had returned to normal and I was not experiencing any rectal bleeding, that meant my inflammation was gone. "This tells me you are all better," he said confidently.

"Um… with all due respect, I'm not," I replied. "I'm still running to the bathroom at least ten, fifteen times a day. I'm still wearing Depends to work and having accidents. I still have this tightness and tenderness in my stomach."

He pointed at the numbers on the screen again. "These numbers here, this is your CRP, C-reactive protein," he said. "This is where you were the last time you were here. Your CRP at that time was 21.72 mg/L, that is very high. Now you are down to 0.18 mg/L, that is a tremendous improvement. This tells me the inflammation is gone." He shrugged, smiled, and said again, "You are all better."

I was very confused.

"Then… why am I still running to the bathroom constantly?" I asked.

"There may be an element of irritable bowel syndrome in addition to the colitis," Dr. Shreck said. "That can be brought on by stress. Your inflammation has gone away. You should consider seeing a psychologist. I believe your problem is all up here," he said, pointing to his head.

On the car on the ride home, Amanda and I had very different reactions to this latest turn of events.

"Hey, this is good news, Russ!" Amanda said encouragingly. "Wouldn't it be great if this really is all in your head?"

"I don't know," I said hesitantly. "First of all, I don't believe that this is just all in my head. But even if it is… I think that might be even worse."

"How so?" Amanda asked, confused.

"Because, I don't know how to…" I fumbled for the words. I didn't know quite how to articulate it, but I tried the best I could. "If it is all in my head, I don't know how to turn it off."

Chapter Twenty-Four

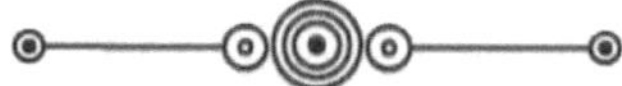

Dr. Shreck telling me that I should see a psychologist lined up with something my parents had been telling me for a while. The stress of everything that I was dealing with was ready to break me. I was trying so hard to find out what could fix me physically that I had been neglecting what all of this was doing to my mental and emotional state.

And while I felt very strongly that my illness was *not* just all in my head, there was certainly a stress component that contributed to it. My colitis added to my anxiety, and my anxiety triggered my colitis. I was trapped in a vicious cycle. Maybe a mental health professional could help me manage it. It was not the worst idea in the world. Even though it would not be a cure for my colitis, if I could add some tools to my toolbox to manage it better, then that was something I shouldn't dismiss out of hand.

A family member had gone through several therapists before he found one who he really connected with and who had helped him a lot. My parents gave me his name and contact info and said I should reach out to him. His name was Dr. Maroni.

I saw Dr. Maroni for the first time in February 2009. He was a tall, older, bald man with a deep baritone voice and an Italian accent.

Of course, I went through the whole sordid story of my disease and everything I had been through. Although I had gotten quite used to it by now, explaining it all to each new doctor or professional honestly never got any easier. For one thing, my natural inclination was always to downplay or downright hide what I was going through. Even in a setting like this, where the whole point of me being there was to talk about everything, it was hard to bring those walls down.

For another thing, there was now so much that I had been through that it was hard to summarize everything. I mean, look how long this book is already. How was I supposed to get someone up to speed on how I got here in one visit?

Dr. Maroni commented that I seemed uncomfortable. I admitted that I was. I said it was hard for me to be out anywhere unfamiliar or away from a bathroom. He told me how to get to the nearest bathroom from his office and that if I needed to use it, I could do so. That was reassuring, but my guard was still up, like I was on edge. But then again, that had pretty much become my natural state.

We walked through some breathing exercises. Dr. Maroni told me to put my hands on my stomach. Most of the time, we all tend to breathe in relatively shallow breaths, especially in times of stress. Dr. Maroni wanted me to breathe in slowly and deeply through my nose to a count of five, really breathing down deep into my stomach so that my belly would fill up like a beach ball. Then I was to hold my breath for another count of five seconds, and then slowly exhale through my mouth to a count of eight. In through the nose, letting my belly fill up like a balloon to a count of five, hold for a count of five, out through the mouth for a count of eight. Repeat. Repeat.

If you have never tried this breathing exercise, you should. It is quite calming.

But after doing it for a few minutes, I thought, *Okay, now what?*

It was a good relaxation technique, but it did not fix anything. I realized as I was sitting there that I was still desperate to just be "better." Breathing exercises were not going to do the trick. I felt like I was back with Dr. Yeardley, waiting for the hypnosis to kick in and put me back into that magical state I had gotten to the first time. The breathing was not relaxing me enough *because* I was thinking about how it was not relaxing me enough.

Dr. Maroni recommended two books that he wanted me to read. But money was too tight, and I had no time to read, so I never got them.

I saw Dr. Maroni every two weeks for a couple of months. Each time, I paid a $25 copay. There was a sign near the reception desk saying that any cancellations must be made at least twenty-four hours in advance. Otherwise, you would still be charged for the session, which would not be billed through insurance, and would cost $200. That sign made me feel more anxious than anything. With how quickly my health could turn on a dime, me not being able to come to a session at the last minute was a very real possibility. Being billed $200 for something I didn't even attend seemed unconscionable.

My financial struggles were the topic of one of my sessions with Dr. Maroni. He asked what kinds of things contributed to my stress, and I said that money was definitely one of them. I said that I worked seven days a week but I never had any money to spend on things that I wanted to spend it on. Even just buying a comic book or a DVD felt like a luxury I couldn't afford when I was struggling to pay all my bills.

Dr. Maroni considered this very thoughtfully for a few moments. Then, in his calm, deep voice, he said, "You plan."

"I'm sorry?" I said.

He spread out his hands as if he were laying something out in front of him. "You must plan. Make a budget. You figure out how much you spend on rent, on bills, on groceries, everything. You add it all up. You see how much is left. And then, you should be able to buy the DVD."

I sat in silence.

After four sessions with Dr. Maroni, I just stopped scheduling them. He never called to ask why I stopped coming or anything. We were just done.

Another side effect of all the medications I was taking and the fact that my immune system was suppressed was that I started developing warts on my hands. This happened gradually. I'd had two or three small ones on my left hand, between my thumb and index finger, shortly before the wedding.

I remember the photographer taking a close-up photo of me and Amanda with our hands together next to the bouquet of flowers, to show our wedding rings, and I consciously shifted my hand in such a way as to make sure to hide the warts. Now, several months later, both of my hands were covered in warts. Big, nasty ones across the backs of my hands near my knuckles, and then smaller ones that went up my fingers. They looked horrific.

When I was at work, I would try to conceal them as best I could. The jacket that I was already wearing every day at 13 WHAM to carry my adult diapers in had really long sleeves. I'd let the sleeves hang down loose and cover most of my hands, so just my fingers from about the second knuckle onward were poking out. I'd be in the studio, gripping the handles of the big studio camera, and I'd have the ends of my sleeves wrapped around most of my hands.

At Sam's Club, it was harder to hide. Granted, I was in a back office behind two locked doors most of the time, but I had to go out to do the cash pulls. That was a process that involved me unlocking each and every cash register and reaching in to take out hundreds of dollars. You'd better believe every cashier was watching my hands very closely as I did that, which meant they were all seeing all my fat ugly warts.

I eventually started wearing fingerless compression gloves to Sam's. Compression gloves are meant to put light pressure and warmth on your hands to help with arthritis or other inflammation or swelling of the hands. For me, they covered up most of my warts, or at least they covered up the worst of them. They didn't conceal the smaller ones that went up my fingers, but at least they hid a decent amount of them.

Of course, now I had to explain why I was wearing the gloves. My manager asked me one time, and I said I had a repetitive stress disorder. She looked worried and said she hoped I was not developing carpal tunnel from working in the cash office. Another time, a coach saw just enough of the redness and small warts creeping out of the top of the glove to ask me, "How did you get those burns?" Rather than say, "Oh, they're not burns, they're warts," I just said, "I don't really want to talk about it." Who knows what he thought my story was.

One day when I was working, there was a call over the walkie-talkie saying that the lines were really long at the cash registers and they needed some help line-rushing if anyone was available. Line-rushing was a process where we could scan someone's membership card with a hand scanner while they were still in line, scan all of their items, and then suspend the order so that when the customer got to the register, the cashier simply had to scan their membership card again and their total would come right up. It was a fast and efficient way to get the lines down in a hurry.

I was caught up on my work in the office at the moment, so I figured what the hey, I'll give them a hand. I grabbed a scanner and emerged from my back-room hiding place and helped knock down the lines.

After the lines were back down to a manageable status, I went back in the cash office, feeling pretty good about myself for doing my good deed for the day. While I was heading back, another associate stopped me to say thank you for helping out. He stuck out his hand for a handshake, and without thinking, I reached out and accepted the handshake. I was not wearing my gloves. He recoiled in horror.

"What's all over your hands?" he gasped.

"Oh," I said, suddenly embarrassed. "Those are just warts."

"Are they contagious?" he asked.

"No," I said, shaking my head quickly, looking down. "No, they're not contagious." Honestly, I had no idea if they were or not. I didn't think they were. I assumed I just had them because of my compromised immune system, but I could not swear to the fact that they weren't contagious.

There was a bottle of hand sanitizer nearby. He immediately squirted a liberal dose of hand sanitizer onto his hands and rubbed it all over vigorously.

"Well, hey, I've got kids at home, y'know?" he said. "I'll just use some of this, and we'll both feel a lot better!" Then he very quickly exited the room.

I went into the cash office, closed the door behind me, and sat down. I just stared at the floor for a while. I was so ashamed. I was practically a leper. That coworker had been absolutely horrified when he saw my hands. As much as I hated having Crohn's, I'd gotten really good at keeping that a secret. There was no hiding the warts. I wanted them to just go away.

At 13 WHAM, in the summer of 2009, a longtime employee in the marketing department announced he was retiring. He edited commercial spots for advertisers as well as promos for the news. He worked the standard nine to five, which seemed like an absolute dream to someone like me who was starting their workday at 3:30 a.m. Plus, this was a full-time position, which meant it came with health benefits, which I, in my perpetual part-time status, did not have.

My wheels started turning immediately. I wanted that job. I knew I was a good editor. How could I prove it? I decided I would take the initiative to make an ad for our morning news show without even being asked, before they even started taking applicants for the job.

Every episode of *13 WHAM News This Morning* was backed up and cataloged on DVD. The DVDs filled up row upon row of binders that were on shelves outside of the edit bays. This way, if we needed to pull footage of something that had aired previously, we could access it quickly. I started using any downtime I had to pull clips from the DVDs. There were a lot of fun celebrity guests that were interviewed via satellite on the morning show in those days. Richard Simmons. Kim Kardashian. Bill Nye the Science Guy. Noah Wyle. Bob Saget. There was even one segment where Evan Dawson interviewed Kermit the Frog and Miss Piggy. I sat in the edit bays and saved any fun, funny clips from those interviews that I could find.

As I was going through these clips of interviews, I decided that just doing one promo was not going to be ambitious enough. So I also started pulling clips from the recurring Soul Plates segment that I mentioned earlier.

Then I went onto the station's shared drive and found the folder where they had all the music beds, the station logo and background animation, and even sound drops of the announcer introducing the show. I saved copies of those for my little project as well.

Once I had this wealth of content at my fingertips, I chipped away at creating not one, not two, but *three* promos. I made a sixty-second version of the celebrity interview highlights; a tighter, faster-paced thirty-second version of the celebrity interviews; and then a thirty-second Soul Plates spot.

I burned all three promos to a DVD. I was proud of how they came out. They were pretty darn good, especially considering I was working from material I had gathered up all on my own. By this time I had spent a couple of weeks of working on these videos during my lunch break, after my shift was over, or any free time I had when I was caught up on my other duties. I was really hoping this would show ambition, resourcefulness, creativity, and above all, how much I wanted the job.

As soon as I had the DVD finished, I tracked down the director of Marketing and Promotion at 13 WHAM in the hallway as I was about to leave for the day. He would have been the one hiring the replacement.

"Hey," I said, very nervous but trying to sound super casual. "Do you have a sec?"

"Sure, what's up?" he replied.

"Um, I was wondering what the plans are for filling the marketing position?"

"Not sure yet," he said. "Definitely have not made any decisions or anything like that."

"All right," I said. "Um, well I'd love to be considered for it." I handed him the DVD. "I put together a few spots for the morning show, just to kind of show my editing skills. I hope you guys will keep me in mind."

"Oh!" He seemed genuinely surprised. He smiled and took the DVD. "I will do that. Thanks a lot."

"Thanks you!" I said. No, that is not a typo. In my nervousness, I said "Thanks you" instead of "Thanks" or "Thank you." I walked away immediately.

A couple of weeks later, they announced that someone else would be taking on the position. I had not gotten an interview, and I received no feedback on my promo DVD. It had never been acknowledged at all after that awkward hallway exchange.

The guy who got the job had been at 13 WHAM a lot longer than me and definitely had more experience. He was a videographer that they would send out on location to shoot everything from sporting events to house fires. Even if I had gotten the interview, it would have been no contest between me and him. It still stung.

I had gotten my hopes up that maybe something better was coming, and it had been for nothing.

But then again, I was getting awfully used to that feeling.

One day at Sam's Club, I was working in the cash office by myself when Coach Bob came in, along with Rick, an associate from the floor who was in training to be a manager. Rick needed to be cross-trained in all the different areas of the Club, and one of the areas he still needed some exposure to was the accounting office.

Coach Bob asked if it would be all right if Rick sat in and shadowed me for a while and I could show him the ropes. I said sure, no problem. I was in the middle of counting a cash pull, which was not the most exciting thing in the world, but it was a pretty good example of what usually went on in that tiny room— counting large amounts of money very carefully.

Rick could not be alone in the accounting office, because only managers or cash office associates were allowed to be in there alone, and he was not yet a manager.

Coach Bob left, and I proceeded to narrate everything I was doing—counting the money, how to bundle it, what to enter into the computer and where to log it, stuff like that.

Then, suddenly and without warning, I felt the strong, urgent sensation in my bowels that let me know that something was going to need to come out imminently.

I didn't know what to do.

Rick had only been in the office with me a few minutes. I was right in the middle of showing him how to count the pull and put it together for the bank deposit. I was not allowed to leave him alone in here. If I was going to leave the room, I would have to say, "I need to go to the bathroom right now." Both of us would have to leave the room, and I would have to set the alarm on the door. There was no way to do this without making it clear to him that I was about to shit my pants.

Also, even if I did do that, I was not confident that I would not, in fact, shit my pants in the process. The time it was going to take to tell Rick we needed to leave the room right now, which was already going to be super awkward, and then actually leave the room, and then for me to set the alarm on the door, and then sprint to the bathroom was most likely not going to be enough time.

So now I am sitting there trying to consider if it's possible to gracefully and discreetly shit my pants. Was there a way that I could actually defecate, in my pants, right there in the cash office, with a coworker sitting right next to me, without him realizing that was what was happening? What were the odds of me pulling that off? I was sitting down in a chair. If I was standing up, *maybe* I could do it. Was there a reason for me to stand up right now? Was there a book or folder or something in the room I could show him that would be relevant to the conversion that I could nonchalantly stand up to go get, and in the process of so doing, casually shit my pants?

What was the better move here? Tell this guy "I need to go to the bathroom" and have him realize I was about to shit my pants, or try to find a way to actually shit my pants and hope he did not realize what I was doing?

Just then, a call came in over the walkie-talkie he had clipped to his belt. "Hey, Rick?" someone asked, followed by the walkie's familiar chirp-like beep.

He took the walkie off of his belt, held in the button and replied.

"Hey, can you come drive the forklift? We need something dropped out of the steel."

Rick sighed and rolled his eyes. "Well, that didn't last long," he said to me. "Guess we'll have to continue this another time. Thanks anyway, Russ." Then, into the walkie-talkie, he said, "Sure, I'll be right out."

He got up and walked over to the door.

I stood up too. For a split second, I was going to say, "I'll walk out with you, I'm going to take a quick bathroom break" or something like that. It seemed more natural now. Rick was getting up to leave, so I could use that as an excuse to basically say *hey, you know what, now that you mention it, I'll walk out, too, and use the restroom.* But as soon as I stood up, I knew this was not going to work. I would not even be able to walk across this small room.

As soon as the door closed behind him, I released the tension I was holding in and soiled myself.

I stood there in complete disbelief of how that had timed out. I was so lucky, I thought. Thank God Rick had gotten that call over the walkie when he did and had to leave the office. What a relief that it had worked out so well. I felt like someone was looking out for me.

Then the absurdity of the moment hit me. I was standing there, having just defecated in my pants, thinking about how lucky I was. Couldn't that someone who was looking out for me have made it so I didn't need to shit my pants at all?

I leaned my head against the wall and laughed like I was losing my mind.

Chapter Twenty-Five

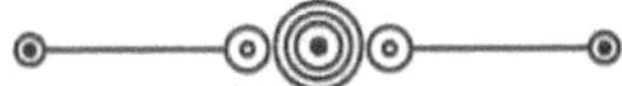

In the fall of 2009, I was back on the three p.m. to midnight shift at 13 WHAM for a bit, filling in for an evening director on vacation. I was on my dinner break after the six o'clock news had ended, and Amanda and I met up at a Panera near the station.

"Hey, there's a new acupuncturist that just started working at the Life Center," Amanda mentioned. The Life Center was where Amanda primarily did her music therapy sessions. They offered many different forms of creative arts therapy there, including art and dance therapy as well. "I talked to her a bit today. Her name is Teagan. Digestive disorders are actually one of her specialties. She has celiac disease herself, so I'm sure she must know a lot about them. Have you thought about giving acupuncture another try?"

"Hmm… not really," I said, dismissively.

"Why not?"

"I don't know. It just feels like one more thing, y'know?"

"Well… I did mention you to her," Amanda said. "So she might be expecting your call." She said it encouragingly with a look of hope in her eyes, but still a bit hesitantly. I think she couldn't tell if she was being helpful or just adding yet another thing to my plate. To be honest, I wasn't sure either.

It was hard each time a new possibility presented itself. I went through a strange combination of getting my hopes up and remaining skeptical at the same time. It seems like a contradiction, but those feelings can occur simultaneously, and it's a stressful way to feel. Also, anything new came with more time commitments and more money to spend. It almost didn't seem worth it. But still. What if this was finally the thing that worked?

"All right," I said. "What could it hurt to call her?"

I made an appointment to meet with Teagan in the second week of September 2009.

At our first meeting, she greeted me excitedly as if we had known each other forever. Some people give off an energy as soon as you meet them that makes you feel like you know them already. This blonde-haired, blue-eyed woman radiated a warm and welcoming energy that made me feel like I was running into an old friend rather than meeting someone for the first time. "Come on back," she said, inviting me into the acupuncture room.

We chatted for a bit. I went over the list, for the umpteenth time, of everything I had already tried for my Crohn's. When I told her I had tried acupuncture once before, she seemed intrigued.

"Really?" she asked. "How did it go for you?"

"I didn't see a whole lot of relief from it," I said. "I found it relaxing. But my symptoms… well… it didn't really do the trick." I thought back to some of my early conversations with Abby. "My previous acupuncturist didn't have experience treating Crohn's, specifically. I don't know if she just didn't know exactly what to do for me or if I didn't give it enough of a chance. Or both."

"Stick out your tongue for me," Teagan said.

I was confused. "For real?" I asked.

"Yes! Didn't your previous acupuncturist ever check your tongue?"

"No…"

She put her hands on her hips. "What kind of acupuncturist doesn't check your tongue?" she said incredulously, with the tone of a new girlfriend who is trying to measure up against your ex. "You can tell all kinds of things about a person's health by looking at their tongue. Go on, let me see."

I stuck my tongue out and said "ahhh." She leaned in a little and examined it closely. I have no idea what she was looking for or what she could tell from my tongue or even if she was just putting me on. She seemed so quirky. I was at ease with her.

"Did you ever try any Chinese herbs with her?" she asked.

"Um, yes, but I don't remember the names of any of them."

"Okay," she said. She was taking notes while we talked. "I'm going to give you some herbs to try, but I'll have to bring them in next time. I don't have them here. I actually have another office that I practice out of. I'm only here at the Life Center two days a week." Then, noticing my hands, she said, "Hey, what's going on here?"

"Oh," I said, instinctively turning my hands away so she couldn't see them. "I have warts."

"Let me see," she said gently.

I showed her my hideous wart-ridden meat hooks.

"Oh, you poor guy," she said sympathetically. She seemed so caring and compassionate from the very first minutes of our visit. "Let me look into some herbs that might help with those too, okay?"

"Sure, that would be awesome," I said.

We went ahead and did an acupuncture treatment that day, which was very similar to my experiences the first time. Teagan asked a few questions about where Abby had put her needles compared to where she was putting hers. It was so funny to me— she almost seemed competitive. I closed my eyes and tried to enjoy the opportunity to relax. I did the breathing exercises I had learned from Dr. Maroni. I even tried to visualize some of the boat imagery that Dr. Yeardley had included in her hypnotherapy routine. I was becoming the sum of a lot of different medical professionals' parts.

As our first session ended, Teagan asked if I would be willing to come to her other office for our next session.

My next appointment with Teagan was at an office in Pittsford, New York. She had some herbs for me: Pulsatilla, Yi Zi Tang, and Di Yu Tan. She explained that the Pulsatilla and Di Yu were key to stopping bleeding at the end of the colon. They were in a powder form to ensure maximum absorbency.

The reason she wanted to see me at her other office was that she wanted to use a kind of Chinese therapy called moxibustion, which involves burning dried mugwort herb. "It smells a little bit like… marijuana." She whispered the last word. "I can't burn it at the Life Center. To be honest, they're not crazy about me burning it here, either. The building owner has a nose like Scooby-Doo. But he's not around today, so let's go for it!"

So round two of acupuncture with Teagan was accompanied by the weed-like smell of moxa. I didn't know if it was helping, but we sure were going into new territory here. I enjoyed my sessions with her and found her enthusiasm to be entertaining. Her bubbly personality was certainly about as far as you could get from the cold bedside manner of Dr. Shreck. At least I was getting some variety now.

Meanwhile, I had to figure out what I was going to do about the warts. I couldn't wait for the day that my Crohn's was in remission and I could get off immune-suppressing drugs because for all I knew, that day might never come. Teagan had said she would look into some herbs for me, but I was getting desperate to get rid of them fast.

I went to see my primary care doctor and asked if there was anything he could do. He said that usually the first step for treating warts would be salicylic acid, and that you can buy that over the counter. Given the number and severity of the warts, though, he suggested we try freezing them, which would be a more aggressive form of treatment.

The doc took out a can of what looked like a big spray can of WD-40 or the compressed air you use to clean dust out of your computer keyboard. It was liquid nitrogen. He sprayed it on the many, many warts that covered the backs of both of my hands. At first it did not really feel that bad, just like cold air. It took about thirty seconds or so for him to spray all of the warts. He told me that throughout the day the skin would get red and irritated and that was normal; essentially, the cryotherapy was triggering the body's natural immune response, and as my skin healed, it would heal the warts as well. I envisioned a bunch of white blood cells showing up to heal my chapped hands, noticing the warts and saying, "Heeeeey! What are these guys doing here?"

As the day went on, the skin on my hands became increasingly irritated and sore. They had that red, raw, blistery look and feel you get if you're outside in the winter without gloves on for too long. They felt itchy all the time. I couldn't help but rub and scratch at them, which only brought my attention back over and over again to how awful they looked. The next day at work, my hands cracked and bled, and it was hard to even move the computer mouse in the edit bay because moving my fingers caused the skin to pull and rip like paper. My hands still looked abominable, and now they hurt like hell on top of it. Couldn't anything ever just give me relief without making me more miserable first?

I went back to the doctor a week later for a follow-up. The warts did not look any better. Mercifully, the doctor did not hit them with another dose of the freezing spray. Although he did say that it sometimes takes multiple administrations of the cryotherapy to have an effect, he now felt that my case was so severe that he wanted to refer me to a dermatologist. I'm not sure why we couldn't have just done that in the first place and spared me from having my mitts turned to what resembled bloody ground beef. He referred me to a dermatologist in Rochester, Dr. Thomas. I made an appointment to get in to see him.

By this point, I was constantly reading up on treatments for Crohn's and colitis, online on message boards, in books, pretty much anywhere I could think to look. My parents would often send me things that they found in magazines or that they had printed out off of websites as well. I could not let go of my sense of feeling like there must be a "magic bullet" out there that we had not found yet, and if we could just find that one thing, it would make me better.

One of the up-and-coming therapies for Crohn's was something called low-dose naltrexone (LDN). Naltrexone was traditionally used as an opiate inhibitor to treat people with drug addictions. It blocks the effects of drugs like morphine and heroin and is used to treat people with addictions to those drugs. There was some research showing that in low doses—about a tenth of the dose typically used for opioid addiction treatment—it could also help reduce inflammation, and it had been successful in some patients in treating multiple sclerosis, fibromyalgia, and Crohn's.

It was an "off-label" prescription, meaning that although the FDA had approved LDN, they had not approved it for Crohn's treatment specifically. It was not an uncommon practice for doctors to prescribe medications off-label as long as there was significant evidence to suggest the drug was safe and effective to use for that condition. I decided I would ask Dr. Shreck about LDN at my next appointment.

As I went into my next appointment, I knew I was going to have to be more assertive. That last visit where he had tried to suggest that it was all in my head had still left a bad taste in my mouth. I knew I was going to have to really convey how bad things still were and get him to understand my situation.

Sure enough, at my next visit Dr. Shreck again raved about how great my CRP numbers were, and that that indicated that my inflammation was way down. Again, like my last appointment, he repeated the phrase, "You are all better."

"But I'm not," I had to insist. "I'm still running to the bathroom, sometimes ten, twelve times a day. I have to wear diapers to work. I get this tight, painful, urgent feeling right here," I said, pointing to my abdomen just below my belly button. "I'm still having accidents. I'm not all better, Dr. Shreck, I'm really not."

"That is the IBS," he said.

I didn't have a super clear definition of what he meant by IBS as opposed to Crohn's. Or colitis, or whatever the hell I had. It may have been a clear distinction in his mind, but it wasn't in mine. All I knew was that I was sick and suffering.

"I think that is stress related," he said. "I think you should consider seeing a psychologist." He turned to Lorraine, who once again was looking at me sympathetically. Obviously she never said so, but I think she was affected by the obvious contrast between what I was saying and how Dr. Shreck was responding to me. Though that could certainly have just been me reading into it. "We have a name of someone, I think? There is a psychologist who specializes in patients with digestive disorders. We have referred patients in the past."

She nodded and began looking through some records on the computer, trying to find the name of the psychologist Dr. Shreck was thinking of.

Amanda was, as always, sitting next to me. She reached over and gently put her hand on my hand. "Hey," she said softly. "Maybe this is a good time to ask about that other medicine you were reading about." She was always good at trying to help prompt me when she knew there was something I wanted to bring up.

"Um, so I have been reading about low-dose naltrexone," I said awkwardly. "It sounds like that has been helpful to a lot of Crohn's patients lately and getting them into remission. Is that something I could try?"

Dr. Shreck looked at me like I had two heads. "LDN is an opiate," he said. "If you take that, you will have colitis, IBS, and a narcotic addiction!"

That made no sense to me. Everything I had read said that naltrexone was an opiate inhibitor, not an opiate. You would have thought I'd just asked him if I could try heroin! But even with all the reading I had done, I didn't feel confident enough or knowledgeable enough to argue with a doctor. I sadly dropped the subject.

Lorraine found the name of the psychologist.

"Dr. Yeardley," she said. "She has been very successful in treating patients with digestive disorders using hypnotherapy. I can give you her phone number."

My heart sank. I slumped forward and ran my hands over my face in frustration. "I've seen her," I said. "I tried her hypnotherapy last year."

"And it didn't help?" Dr. Shreck said, sounding shocked. Something about him being surprised that hypnotherapy had not helped me was funny and infuriating at the same time.

I shook my head. "It helped a little, at first, but…" I gestured to myself and then to the room we were in, as if to say, *If it had helped, would we be here right now?*

Dr. Shreck looked thoughtful for a moment. Then he said, "I am going to prescribe you a medication called Bentyl." He began writing. "It is an anti-spasmodic. It will help with the urgency you feel."

I couldn't believe it.

"We already tried that," I said. There was an anger in my voice that I had never used in speaking to a doctor before.

He looked up from his notes. "And what happened?" he said, surprised.

"At first it helped a lot," I said.

Dr. Shreck smiled, as if to say, *See?*

"But then I started to have a rebound effect. The medication would help for a shorter and shorter time, each time. And every time the urgency came back, it got worse and worse. It was like everything was building up. Like the periods of relief just added up to more symptoms later on." I couldn't believe I was having to explain this again after we had already gone over it two visits ago.

After a moment, Dr. Shreck went back to writing in his notebook. "I would like you to try it again," he said. "Give it another chance. I think this will get your IBS symptoms under control."

I was seething. Why would I try it again after what happened last time? I didn't want to go through that again. The periods of relief that I got initially were not worth the suffering that came later. That New Year's Eve that I spent on the toilet was not something I could relive. I just couldn't subject myself to that again just because Dr. Shreck was out of other ideas. I was so mad I felt like I could scream. I was clenching my fists. I wanted to punch him.

"Do you want me to write out the prescription, or we can send it right to the pharmacy?" he asked.

"Neither," I said. I was livid.

He looked up again, surprised.

"I'm not taking that again," I said. My voice was controlled but filled with anger and disgust. I wasn't yelling; I was quietly pissed off, which I think was probably scarier. "It didn't work last time, and I told you that. I ended up with worse symptoms. It was horrible. I am not putting myself through that again, so don't bother writing the prescription."

He laughed. He looked at me, then at Amanda, then at Lorraine. He shook his head. "There is something else going on here," he said. "This is stress related. You must see a psychologist," he said. His tone was extremely condescending. As far as he was concerned, me getting angry and pushing back against his advice was proving his point that I was having mental problems. He looked at Amanda, then said, again, "He must see a psychologist." As if he was telling her that she needed to make sure I got some mental help.

I didn't say anything else. I was two seconds away from completely losing it. I wish I had said, *If you want to know why I'm stressed, it's because I'm shitting my pants every day while you tell me I'm all better, asshole!* I wish I would have yelled it loud enough for all the other patients to hear. I wish I had called him a quack and said I was never coming here again, then stormed out of the building ranting and raving and making a scene. *You think I need a psychologist? I'll show you how crazy I am! They can take me out of your office in a goddamn straitjacket!*

But I didn't do that. I felt like if I wigged out, I would have just been proving him right.

I put a lid on my boiling pot of anger and let it simmer instead of spilling over.

One thing I was sure of, though. I was never seeing him again.

It was time, yet again, to find another doctor.

Chapter Twenty-Six

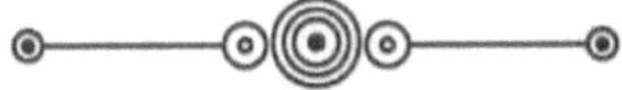

At the next support group meeting, I told everyone about the latest escapade with Dr. Shreck. I didn't use his name of course, as per the rules of the group, so I had to just refer to him as "my doctor."

Everyone was aghast at the story—at how he had tried to get me back on a medication that I'd had a bad experience with, how he'd continued to suggest that this was somehow all in my head, and how he'd dismissed LDN and said it would just lead to me having a narcotic addiction. Everyone in the group seemed truly horrified at hearing all of this. I said I felt like I needed to stop seeing him and find a new doctor, but that I was also so exhausted and discouraged at the prospect of having to, once again, try to find someone else and start all over.

"Russ, can you and Amanda stay for a few minutes after the group is over?" Betty asked. "I want to talk to you a little more about this."

"Sure," I said.

After the meeting, Amanda and I stuck around to talk to Brian and Betty.

"So, as you know, as the leader of the support group I can't ask you this," Betty said. "So I am asking you this as a fellow Crohn's patient and as a friend." I felt like we were trying to get around the first two rules of Fight Club. "If you are comfortable telling me, who is the doctor that you're seeing now?"

Of course I was comfortable telling her. "His name is Dr. Shreck," I said.

Betty did not seem surprised. In fact, she seemed annoyed. "You are not the first to have that kind of experience with him, I'm sorry to say," she said. "I have heard stories about him from other patients as well, saying that he just doesn't listen to them or is very short and abrupt with them."

I wish this could have been brought to my attention sooner.

I sighed. "Okay, well, I guess I'm glad it's not just me," I said. It did make me feel like at least I wasn't crazy.

"I do think that changing doctors is the right next step for you," Betty said. "I know how hard it is to start all over with someone new. But the lack of concern and respect he is showing you is unacceptable."

I hadn't thought about it that way, but when she said it, I knew she had hit the nail on the head. I needed a doctor who cared more about my well-being than about being right. Dr. Shreck was not it.

"I have run this support group for twenty years," she continued. "I have seen people who are the victims of stress and truly are their own worst enemy. But Russ, I don't see you that way at all. I don't think your doctor is giving you enough credit for what you have been through."

I felt empowered by what she said. With a renewed sense of purpose, I went back to the drawing board and started researching GI doctors in the area yet again.

One name that kept coming up in my searches was Dr. Calvin, a doctor who was affiliated with Rochester General Hospital. I was part of a listserv that discussed Crohn's and colitis treatments, and LDN had been a hot topic as of late. Since it was an off-label prescription, not every GI doctor would prescribe it. (Boy, we sure learned that, didn't we?) Someone had collected a list of doctors who had prescribed it, and Dr. Calvin was on the list. Not that I wanted to choose a doctor based solely on that, but it was good to know. Also, thinking back to my conversation with the contact from the CCFA, Dr. Calvin was the other name he had given me besides Dr. Shreck. His first pick hadn't worked out so well for me, but there was no way he could be wrong about both of them… right?

I reached out to Dr. Calvin's office to see if I could get in to see him for a second opinion. Although, I guess technically this would be a fourth opinion. The soonest they could get me in was May. It was February. I was going to have to try to hang in there for a few more months before I would even be able to see this guy.

At the suggestion of my parents, Amanda and I had cooled off the house hunt for a while after that last place we had looked at back in January. However, in 2009, President Obama had instituted the first-time homebuyers' tax credit. If you bought a house between January 1 and December 1, 2009, you would receive a credit for 10% of the purchase price, up to $8,000. Since our lease on the apartment would be up in May and we were thinking of buying a house anyway, it seemed crazy not to try to do it now.

With the weather starting to turn a little nicer and more houses coming on the market, we began looking at some houses again with Funcle Al. We tried to have an attitude of, *When we see the right place, we will know it.* If we didn't find a place, we weren't completely opposed to staying in the apartment for another year… but the idea of leaving that $8,000 on the table was definitely in the back of our minds.

Amanda and I both worked in the Henrietta area during the week, and the Sam's Club I worked at was in Greece, so we primarily looked in those two towns. There was also a listing that came up in Hamlin, which was about ten minutes or so from where my parents lived in Hilton. It was in our price range, so we decided it would not hurt to have a look at it. This would have been a farther commute for both of us—Hamlin was probably thirty or forty minutes away from Henrietta.

Well, wouldn't you know, we looked at the Hamlin house and both fell in love with it. It was on a quiet little street in a housing tract that reminded both of us of where we had each grown up. It was a split-level, with a quaint living room and a kitchen that had lots of sunlight coming in to illuminate all of the many white cabinets, cupboards, and drawers. Down one level was a bonus room that would be just perfect for an office, plenty of storage, and a laundry room with a half bath. Up one level were three bedrooms and a full bathroom. The backyard was fenced in and had a huge shed in the back for more storage. Best of all, the property backed up to a huge, wide-open green space that would never be built on. It would be a great place for kids to run around and play.

Kids. That was something else to think about. It was not anything we had talked very much about, but we were married and close to buying a house… that was what came next, right?

But how could I possibly be a dad in my current condition? Was I going to be changing two sets of diapers—mine and the baby's? What was I supposed to do if I was out at the store or the playground or something with the kid and I had to run to the bathroom? I could barely take care of myself right now. How was I going to take care of a child?

But that was a discussion for another day. Right now, we had to talk about the house. We both loved it. We looked at each other and could see it in each other's eyes.

"Damn it!" Amanda exclaimed. "I didn't want to like this one!"

We both laughed. This house made the least sense of any we had looked at in terms of the commute we would have to work. We had gotten spoiled living at the apartment in Chili, which was only about ten or fifteen minutes away from our respective places of employment. We would be trading that quick jaunt in for a commute of at least half an hour on a good day. But there was just something about this house. We had said that when we found the right place, we would know it. And we knew it. This house was meant to be our home.

We put in an offer, and it was accepted. We were homeowners!

Next, it was time to see the dermatologist. His office was in Rochester, in another complex of similar-looking medical office buildings that reminded me a bit of where we had gone to see Dr. Shreck. Dr. Thomas had a big bushy mustache, and he reminded me of Dr. Jinga Janga, the genie-ologist who treated Jambi the Genie when he got sick in an episode of *Pee-Wee's Playhouse*. The warts on my hands were as bad as they had ever been; the cryo treatment had done nothing except irritate my skin and make me more uncomfortable. I had also developed warts on the bottom of my feet. I didn't care about those as much since no one could see them.

Dr. Thomas said that he would treat the warts with a laser. This sounded great to me. I envisioned him zapping them and the warts just disappearing, like he was blasting them off. He cautioned me that the laser would be painful, especially given the number of warts that I had. I honestly didn't care. I just wanted these little bastards gone. I didn't care what it felt like at this point.

Dr. Thomas left, and then a nurse came in to do the procedure. The laser was a small handheld device about the size and shape of a tool that a dentist might use to clean your teeth. It was connected via a cable to a larger device with a computer screen where the nurse adjusted the settings. The nurse warned me again that it would hurt. I thought, *How bad could it be?*

She held the laser over my hand and started going over each wart one by one. It made a sort of *pzz-ink, pzz-ink, pzz-ink* noise as it released a little pulse of light over each one. It did not feel anything like I thought it was going to feel. Like being jabbed by a needle, and I don't mean the gentle acupuncture needles. It felt like someone was taking a syringe and stabbing it into my sensitive hands over and over. I looked up at the ceiling and tried to do my slow breathing and think of something else, anything else. It wasn't working. Each jab brought my focus right back to my hands, to say nothing of the soldering iron-like smell of my own burning flesh that filled my nostrils.

When she did the bottom of my feet, that was even worse. It felt like my feet were being carved up for Thanksgiving dinner. I instinctively closed my eyes and held my breath.

"Don't do that," the nurse said suddenly. "Don't hold your breath. You're going to pass out. Try to breathe through it. Do you need to take a break?"

"No," I said. "Just keep going." I didn't want this to take any longer than it had to. I tried to just breathe naturally, but it was like I forgot how to. Do I breathe in, and then out? There was no rhythm to my breathing. I was taking short, shallow, panic breaths as I was stabbed in the soles repeatedly. The room was turning red.

"All done," the nurse said after what felt like forever. "Your hands and feet will feel sore for a few days. We will need to see you back in a couple of weeks to do this again. It will probably take several treatments to get all of them."

I walked out the office tenderly, each footstep feeling like I had broken glass in my soles.

I went back for more laser treatments every couple of weeks. As painful as they were, they at least were working. The skin on my hands and feet turned red and irritated but not nearly as bad as they had been with the cryotherapy. And little by little, the warts started to disappear. Finally, something I was doing was actually working. It was worth putting up with the pain if I was actually going to get somewhere.

One day, I was at work at 13 WHAM in one of the edit bays, and one of the other production guys stopped in to chat.

"Hey, they're looking a lot better," he said.

"Hmm?"

"The warts," he said, nodding toward my hands. "They look a lot better."

"Oh," I said sheepishly. "Yeah, I've been getting a laser treatment on them."

I had somehow let myself think that maybe no one had noticed the warts. I always wore my jacket sleeves to cover them as much as possible, so I'd hoped that maybe they'd gone unseen by my coworkers. I know he was just trying to acknowledge the improvement, but this was the first time anyone there had acknowledged them at all. The first time I knew for sure that they had been noticed.

Another day, I was in sub-control, filling in as the AD for the morning show. It was a role I enjoyed. It was less responsibility than being the director, but still more interactive, and it offered more variety than being in the studio. You got to cue up a lot of the graphics, animations, and videos that were used throughout the newscast from various different sources and make them available for the director to use when he or she needed them.

We went to a commercial break. As I often did, I popped out of sub-control—the AD's seat is conveniently located right next to the doorway into the pit—and made a quick dash to the small bathroom nearby. When I came back, the guy who was directing that day asked the question I had been dreading that someone would one day ask.

"Hey, where do you go when you disappear like that?" he asked.

"What do you mean?" I asked innocently.

"During the commercial breaks, you leave for a minute and then come back. You leave the studio, you leave sub-control. Where the heck are you going?"

"Uh, I don't know!" I said, acting like I had never noticed that I always did that. I was trying not to turn red.

"He's not going to the vending machine," the audio engineer offered. "He never comes back with any snacks or anything."

I laughed as if it was some big joke. "Come on, you guys!" I said, like they were just pulling my leg.

"No, for real, I'm asking." The director was not content to drop it. "Where do you go?"

"I don't know, I just walk around, stretch my legs," I said. It did not sound convincing at all.

"Are you going to the bathroom all the time?" he asked.

"I don't know," I said. "Sometimes that's probably what I'm doing, yeah." I said it like I was speculating as much as they were.

"Jeez. You've got the bladder of an infant, man!"

Yes, that's it. I have the bladder of an infant. Every time I am running out to the bathroom, I'm going to pee. If that's what they wanted to think, that was fine with me. Could you imagine if they knew the truth? Hey, guys, every time that I disappear for a minute or two, I am actually very quickly taking a dump and trying to get back to work as fast as I possibly can, because my intestines are very inflamed all of the time and I have a lot of stool in my colon. But don't worry, I'm also wearing an adult diaper for all of the times that I can't make it in time, which happens almost every day, even with how often you see me running to the bathroom. Wild, isn't it?

Seriously, though, what must everyone be thinking? I had that same sinking feeling I'd gotten back in Virginia at Walmart when I'd been asked if I drink a lot of beer. It revealed that everyone had been talking about me and wondering what was going on. How long could I keep this up before the truth came out? Would something eventually happen where I could not hide my secret anymore?

Months passed. I finally got in for my initial consultation with gastroenterologist Dr. Calvin in mid-May 2009. Amanda came with me, of course, showing her support as always and wanting to make sure that things got off to a good start with the new doctor.

Dr. Calvin walked into the room and immediately gave off a completely different vibe than Dr. Shreck, Dr. Griswold, or Dr. Harvey. He wore a pair of jeans and a button-down shirt. He pulled up a chair and sat right down with us. He had a relaxed demeanor that made me feel like I was talking to a friend.

Of course, I went into the whole story of everything I had been through and everything I had tried so far. He took notes and nodded as I talked. He didn't try to rush us at all. In fact, based on the amount of time he spent with us, you would have thought I was his only patient. I'd had all of my previous records sent over ahead of time, and he had obviously read them over enough to be familiar with my case before we even came in.

At this point I was on Pentasa, Humira, prednisone, and the Cortenema. I had been on 6-MP for a while with Dr. Griswold, but Dr. Shreck had discontinued it.

"All right, I want to try to get you off of the prednisone as soon as possible," Dr. Calvin said. "That's a nasty thing to stay on for a long time. I know you've tried a few times already, but let's start trying to taper you off of it again. If the taper fails and you start to flare up again, we have some other things we can try. We can revisit the 6-MP, or we may consider methotrexate. I would also reconsider the benefit of keeping you on the Humira if the prednisone taper fails, because that should really be keeping you in remission by now with how long you've been on it." He paused for a moment. "Or should I say, it should have gotten you into remission by now." He gestured to the thick stack of records that I'd had sent over from my other doctors. "Russ, I don't think you've been in remission at all since you were diagnosed."

As soon as I heard those words, there was the stinging sensation of tears forming at the corner of my eyes. No one had ever come out and said that, but it was true. I hadn't. And even just hearing him acknowledge that, hearing a doctor come out and say that I had been fighting this disease without a break this entire time, felt like a weight off of my shoulders. This guy got it. I felt seen.

We also talked about how my diagnosis had changed from Crohn's disease to ulcerative colitis. Dr. Calvin acknowledged that the original findings by Dr. Harvey looked more like Crohn's, but the more recent exam by Dr. Shreck did look more like colitis. He said that, for right now at least, which one it truly was wasn't as important as getting me feeling better, and that we would revisit the diagnosis a little further down the road.

He mentioned a test called a Prometheus test that could help distinguish the two illnesses from one another. He didn't feel that was something we needed to do right away but that we would get to it. This made sense to me. I was fine with putting that piece of the puzzle on the back burner for the time being, as long as we were not outright dismissing it like Dr. Shreck had.

"A couple of other things. Are you on any kind of multivitamin or calcium supplement at all?" he asked.

"No," I said.

"Corticosteroids can lead to bone density loss. Given your long history of being on them, you're at risk for osteoporosis," he explained. "I want to start you on a calcium supplement and a vitamin D supplement."

Great, I thought, something else to worry about. But I appreciated that he was looking out for something that none of the other doctors had even mentioned. Still, it made me think. As hard as it was for me to get through my day, who knew what long-term side effects I was looking at from being on all of these medications? It was something I had to push aside mentally, at least for now.

Amanda and I left that appointment feeling optimistic. The way Dr. Calvin had been so patient and kind, the way he had really listened and responded to us, was so refreshing. I was hesitant to really get my hopes up, but now it felt like we at least had someone else on our side.

Chapter Twenty-Seven

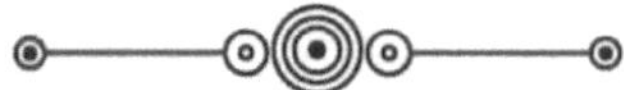

Since the Humira had not worked to get me into remission, Dr. Calvin suggested we discontinue that and try something else. The next drug we were going to try was called Cimzia. It is another biologic agent that you inject yourself with and is often used to treat Crohn's disease and arthritis.

Unlike Humira, Cimzia does not come in a "pen." It's an actual syringe. You have to pinch a hunk of skin on your abdomen, stick the needle into your skin, and slowly press down the plunger. I hated it. I am not a wimp about needles or anything, but pushing a button on the back of a glorified marker that was up against my skin and actually sticking a syringe into myself were two very different things, and this did not feel like a step up.

The injection site would almost always bleed afterward, and it was always a lot sorer than it had been with the Humira. I didn't know if I was doing it wrong or if it was just the nature of the different kind of injection. I came to dread the day every two weeks when I would have to give myself the Cimzia, and based on everything else, I did not even have any hope that it was going to help me.

In the summer of 2009, Dr. Calvin wanted to do another colonoscopy. This would be my fourth. I was starting to wonder if I could get a punch card and eventually get one for free.

One piece of advice I got from the support group in regard to the prep really paid off, and that was to get some Calmoseptine, an ointment to treat and prevent skin irritation. How does that relate to the colonoscopy prep, you ask? Have you ever had a baby with diaper rash? You know how you put Desitin on it to soothe the irritation? Same concept.

When you are going and wiping and going and wiping and going and wiping for hours on end, you wind up with irritated skin. It gets to the point that each time you go, it burns like hell. So not only are you feeling nauseous and glued to the toilet bowl as you clean out everything from your digestive tract, but it also stings like a bitch as it's coming out. So, between episodes, you can apply Calmoseptine down there to soothe it and take one of those awful factors out of the equation. Thanks, support group!

I was unconscious for the whole colonoscopy. I woke up in the "tequila haze" again, reveling in the carefree bliss that it temporarily brought. How ironic that the rare time I could feel truly peaceful was after having my bowels evacuated and explored by a medical professional.

One day at Sam's Club, I noticed a flyer on the bulletin board in the breakroom about a Walmart Community Grant. This was a program where Walmart and Sam's Club gave back to the community by offering funding to nonprofit organizations. All you had to do was fill out an application and write a short essay about why the organization you were nominating deserved the money.

The timing of this was great, as my family and I were once again raising funds for the annual CCFA walk. They had changed their name from "Guts and Glory" to "Take Steps," which disappointed me. You can "take steps" for any charity. I'd loved that the original name had the word "guts" in it.

I no longer have the essay that I wrote, but I really laid all the cards on the table. This essay was going to be read by someone at corporate, not anyone I actually worked with or saw in person, so I didn't hold back. I wrote about how I'd been suffering from Crohn's disease for several years now—I still tended to refer to my illness as Crohn's disease, even though it was possibly colitis—and how I hoped so badly that the funds raised by the CCFA would lead to one day finding a cure for millions of people like me. I also mentioned how the support groups had been an invaluable source of encouragement for me and my wife, and how my family and I did the walk together every year. I even sucked up a little and said how supportive Sam's Club had been with my work schedule, and that Coach John had visited me in the hospital when I was sick. I didn't mention that it was because he had to give me my eval.

My words worked. I received a reply from the Walmart home office in Bentonville, Arkansas, saying they were going to award the CCFA with a grant in the amount of $1,000! I couldn't believe it. I was happy and excited that my essay had gotten us the grant money. This would be huge for our Crohn's Busters team for the fundraiser. The fact I had accomplished that with the power of my own written words meant so much to me.

There was more. A representative from the Walmart home office wanted to come present a check to the CCFA at the morning meeting at my own local Sam's Club, so that I could be there for it. Oops. So much for this just being between me and corporate. Now this was going to be shared with everyone I worked with! This made me nervous.

At a morning meeting at Sam's Club some weeks later, my mom and I and a representative from the CCFA named Stacy went in to accept a huge, oversized, Publisher's Clearing House–looking check in the amount of $1,000 from a member of the Walmart home office. We were all seated in the café area along with all of my morning coworkers, about half an hour before the club opened to the public. Coach Bob and some of the other managers were there too. I asked Stacy if she would be the one to go up and accept the check. She said it should be me, since I wrote the essay. I asked if we could go up together. She said sure.

When it was time go up and accept the check, Stacy stayed seated, and I ended up going up by myself! Everyone was applauding, and I didn't notice that she wasn't with me until I got all the way up to the front. As I stood in front of my colleagues to accept the check, I felt a strange mixture of embarrassment and pride. Coach Bob asked me if I wanted to say a few words.

"I appreciate this very much," I said. "And I'm proud to work for a company that gives back to the community like this. The

Crohn's and Colitis Foundation is a cause that is near and dear to my heart…" I had not planned on saying any of this. It was just tumbling out. "…because I have Crohn's disease myself."

There. I'd said it. If there was ever going to be a time to "come out" to all of my coworkers about having this disease, it was now, when I had just won a thousand dollars from the company we all worked for.

"For those who don't know, Crohn's is an autoimmune disorder that causes your immune system to overreact and start attacking your own digestive system. It causes a lot of inflammation, and it can be very painful. It's been a difficult road for me. I have been in and out of the hospital with flare-ups. I feel sick a lot. And there is no cure. But I hope that one day maybe we can find one, and a contribution like this goes a long way to making that happen. So thank you very much."

Everyone applauded again. I took the big check and walked back over to Stacy and my mom. I gave the check to Stacy along with a look to say, *What the heck, why didn't you come up there with me?*

"See? I told you that you should be the one to accept it," she said. "That was amazing! Everything you said was perfect!"

I felt vulnerable but empowered at the same time. I had shared my secret with a big group of people and nothing bad had happened. In fact, my words had done something for the cause. Maybe it was time to stop hiding in the background all the time. For the first time ever, it occurred to me that maybe my story could help others.

It also gave me the confidence to do one more thing that was long overdue. The next chance I got, I had a talk with the manager of the cash office. I told her that my health had not been in a good place for a long time. I explained that I had been working seven days a week at two jobs for years and that I was beyond burnt out. I asked her if she thought it would be okay if I went down to just working one day a week, either Saturday or Sunday but not both.

She did not even hesitate. "Russ, that would be no problem at all. You need to take care of yourself. Your health has to come first. I'll start scheduling you one day a week."

I had been convinced for so long that if I ever asked to go down to just one day, they would decide they didn't need me and fire me. Until this moment, I had never even thought to try just asking nicely for what I needed.

I would now be working only six days a week, five days at 13 WHAM and one at Sam's Club, with one day off every week. It was a huge step in the right direction for finding a way to take care of myself, and I don't just mean having that day off.

I was finally learning to speak up for myself.

Chapter Twenty-Eight

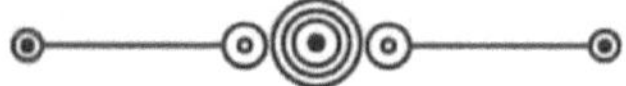

In October, I was back filling in on the three p.m. to midnight shift at 13 WHAM. Amanda and I met up for my dinner break at Panera. I got a plain bagel and a cup of hot tea. I had emailed Dr. Calvin earlier in the day to tell him my symptoms were really acting up again as we tried tapering me off the prednisone—I was back to having blood in my stool and sharp pain in my abdomen. He had emailed me back and asked for a phone number where he could reach me and if he could call me that evening. As Amanda and I were sitting down to eat, my cell phone rang. It was Dr. Calvin.

I felt bad sitting and talking on my phone while Amanda was just sitting there, but she urged me to take it and reassured me that it was fine. I took the call, and Dr. Calvin and I ended up talking for close to half an hour. I was in disbelief that he took the time at the end of his day—it was like seven p.m. at that point— to talk to me for so long. No office visit, no charge, just calling me on his own time to talk about how I was doing and what our next steps should be. It was at this point that he said he felt that surgery was our next step.

He talked about how Crohn's and colitis slowly eat away at your quality of life so much that you get to a point where you don't even realize how limited you've become and how much you've lost. And that statement really hit home.

He was absolutely right. I never hung out with my friends anymore. I didn't enjoy eating. Mealtime was a necessity that I had to force myself through. I had no energy. I felt awful all the time, and any time I left my house, I had to be aware of where the nearest restroom was and how quickly I could get to it. I was wearing adult diapers everywhere I went because I was incontinent.

And as I sat there looking at my dinner of a plain bagel and a cup of tea, listening to my gastroenterologist telling me on his own time how this surgery could get me my life back, that was the moment I really started to think that this might be the right path for me.

Dr. Calvin gave me the name of a colorectal surgeon that he had worked with many times over the years and who he recommended and trusted: Dr. Stevens. He suggested I set up a consultation with him to talk about the possibility of surgery and at least get all the information I could and ask him any questions I had.

Meanwhile, there were some other wheels going into motion. My dad had been working in the handbooks department of a payroll company for several years. One day in November, I got an email from him about a job opening in their Time and Attendance Department. While this was not exactly in my field of expertise, my experience working in the accounting office at Sam's Club was at least something. Plus I was good with computers, was organized, and paid attention to details. This was a full-time, Monday-through-Friday desk job with decent pay and benefits.

I had been waiting around hoping for something full time to open up at 13 WHAM for years now. Maybe it was time to stop waiting. If something was going to change, maybe I would have to make a change. I updated my resume and applied for the position.

In November, I was scheduled for a sigmoidoscopy and consultation with Dr. Stevens to talk about the possibility of surgery. A sigmoidoscopy is kind of like a colonoscopy but much less invasive; they stick a flexible scope into the rectum and the lower part of the large intestine. Unlike a colonoscopy, you are not sedated during a sigmoidoscopy. I didn't even have the "tequila haze" to look forward to this time!

Kind of like the colonoscopy, though, they recommended a liquid diet the day before the procedure, and you had to do a Fleet enema the morning of to "clean out" your rectum. Not as thorough as something like a GoLYTELY or MoviPrep, and I wouldn't be glued to the bowl for the day.

Amanda and I both took the day off from work so she could come with me. It was nice to be able to sleep in a little bit compared to my usual weekday morning wake-up time. I did the

Fleet enema, got out as much as I could, and tried to just relax. I was a bit nervous about the sigmoidoscopy, to be honest. Even though I knew it was not going to be as invasive as a colonoscopy, what if having something stuck up there made me have to go? I'd only had liquids for the last twenty-four hours, but that didn't mean that any stimulation down there wasn't going to trigger something. What if I had an accident during the procedure? Was that something that ever happened?

As we were getting ready to leave the house, I got a phone call. It was the doctor's office. Dr. Stevens had been called into emergency surgery. They were going to have to reschedule my appointment.

I couldn't freaking believe it. I had taken the day off from work—unpaid, of course. I'd gone a whole day without eating anything. I had gone out and bought a Fleet enema and already used it. All for nothing.

They were able to get me in for the following afternoon. Amanda was not going to be able to go with me now because she could not take another day off of work, so I would have to go all by myself. I knew I should probably just keep doing liquids and not eat anything for another day, but I was ravenous. I made a couple of Eggo waffles and rage-devoured them. Then I felt guilty about having eaten something. And on top of all that, I was going to have to go back to the store and buy another Fleet enema.

Amanda, as always, tried to get me to look on the bright side. Now I had a whole day off and didn't have to go anywhere, I could rest, relax, watch TV, just have a "self-care" day. It was hard for me to look at it that way. I just felt like the day was wasted. It made me feel like I wasn't being taken seriously. Sure, logically, I knew that whatever emergency surgery the doctor got called into was probably a pretty bad situation, and I should count myself as lucky that I wasn't on the receiving end of whatever that was. But I couldn't help but feel slighted that I had been "bumped" for something else more important. To me, this was everything. Finding a way to get my health back, and possibly having a major operation to do so, was my life right now. Getting bumped a day, even for a valid reason, was almost too much for me to handle. I was losing my will to keep fighting.

I thought of an old Peanuts comic strip that really resonated with me. Lucy, furious at her family about something, storms across the house and yells, "I GIVE UP!!" In the next panel, Linus, looking confused, says, "Where do you go to give up?" This was how I felt. I was ready to give up, but I did not even know how to do that.

I called my parents and told them what had happened, since they were waiting on news about how my appointment went. When my dad heard that I was going to go by myself, he asked if I wanted him to come with me. I said yes.

The next day, my dad and I went to the appointment at Dr. Stevens's office. Dr. Stevens apologized for having to reschedule me from the day before. He had a calm, matter-of-fact, and professional demeanor, and he spoke in an even tone that was quiet yet confident. He gave off the vibe of someone who had been doing this a long time and was very knowledgeable. The way he spoke kind of reminded me of Dr. Manhattan in the movie *Watchmen.*

Once we had made our introductions, my dad stepped out of the room so Dr. Stevens could perform the sigmoidoscopy. The doctor had me bend over the exam table and drop my pants, and then he inserted a lubricated scope up my butt. I tried to just relax, but it was extremely uncomfortable. In fact, it downright hurt. I grunted and tried to just deal with it, but it really felt unpleasant and intense. I was wincing and felt my whole body clenching and tensing up.

"Is that uncomfortable?" Dr. Stevens asked.

"Yeah," I replied. I was trying to stay composed, but I was whimpering at this point. The scope going up into that sore, sensitive area was killing me.

"All right, I'm going to withdraw the scope," Dr. Stevens said. He carefully removed it. "Take a moment to get your pants back on. I'm going to go bring your dad back in. I'd like to discuss what I've just seen as well as our surgical options."

He left the room. I sighed. Was that supposed to hurt so much? That was really rough. I pulled up my underwear and pants.

My dad came in and he, Dr. Stevens, and I sat down.

"What I just saw, very briefly, on the sigmoid scope was that your rectum is very inflamed," Dr. Stevens stated matter-of-factly. "Normally I would have gone a little farther to examine the lower part of the colon as well, but I could tell you were in a lot of discomfort due to how sensitive and irritated the area was. It did not seem to make sense to proceed any farther when it's so apparent that the disease is present at the very end of your digestive tract."

I nodded. I appreciated that he hadn't tried to "scope up" any farther than he had to. I also felt a little better knowing that the reason it had hurt so much was because of how bad a state my rectum was in. I guess it felt validating in a way.

"Let's discuss surgical options," Dr. Stevens continued. "If I had seen with the scope that your rectum was fine, and the disease was occurring farther up in your colon or if it were in the small intestine, then we might have been able to do a resectioning, where we remove the diseased area and essentially reattach what remains. In that case, we would have been able to preserve your rectum, and you would still go the bathroom normally. Based on what I just saw, that is not an option for you. We would instead want to proceed with a total proctocolectomy with ileostomy surgery.

"What this means is, you would be put under general anesthesia and we would go in laparoscopically and remove the colon and rectum. We would bring the very end of the small bowel, the ileum, out through an opening in your abdomen. This is called a stoma. You would wear an ostomy bag over the stoma to collect waste, rather than going to the bathroom normally when it comes to moving your bowels. Does this make sense?"

"Yes," I said stoically.

This was more or less what I was expecting to hear. I knew that first option, where we would just reattach things and keep the rectum, was out of the question. I thought back to that appointment with Dr. Griswold where I had thought that kind of surgery might be on the table, and how he had explained why it wasn't. I thought about how he had said that the only surgical option for me would be one that resulted in an ostomy bag. *You'd have an ostomy bag for the rest of your life. It doesn't make sense to do something that extreme here*, Dr. Griswold had said at the time. Here we were, a year and a half later, and it was looking more and more like this was the only option left.

Dr. Stevens went on to discuss more details about the potential procedure. I would do a bowel prep ahead of time, similar to what I did before each colonoscopy. At least that was old hat for me at this point. The recovery in the hospital after the surgery was usually about three to seven days, followed by about a month of recovery at home. This period would come with restrictions, such as no driving, no lifting more than ten pounds, and I would once again be on a low-fiber diet—no fresh fruits or veggies, no nuts or popcorn. This all sounded reasonable.

Then he went over the risks of the procedure. I could experience excessive bleeding during the surgery and require a blood transfusion. There was also the risk of infection, either to the wounds from the surgery, the urinary tract, or an abscess of some kind. There was the risk of a blood clot after the surgery. There was the risk that I could have a bad reaction to the anesthesia and have a heart attack or a stroke.

And last but not least, there was the risk of damage to any of the organs or nerves that were near the surgical site. He mentioned very specifically that the nerves that control the male ability to have an erection and ejaculate are right next to where we would be cutting. If those nerves were accidentally nicked during the surgery, there was the possibility that I might not be able to have an erection or ejaculate anymore.

My dad looked over at me to see how I was holding up through all of this. I had been okay until we got to that last possible complication. This surgery was supposed to help me get my quality of life back, and then maybe Amanda and I could start talking about having kids. What if that same procedure made that impossible?

"Um, that last thing that you mentioned," I said. "What are the chances of that happening?"

"The odds of any of these complications arising are small. But I can't promise you that any of them won't happen. I'm just informing you of the possibilities so you can make an informed decision."

I understood that he was just trying to cover all of the bases. Of course he couldn't say, "But this won't happen to you." Because what if it did? We'd seen I was quite good at defying the odds in the things-going-wrong category.

There were additional possible complications for after the surgery, and these were all considered "lifetime risks." Hernia. Obstruction of the ostomy. And a recurrence of Crohn's.

"I understand there is some question about whether you have Crohn's disease or ulcerative colitis," Dr. Stevens said. "If you have colitis, this surgery is a cure. Colitis does not occur anywhere other than the colon and rectum. We are removing those, so you would have no risk of the disease coming back. Crohn's disease, however, can occur anywhere in the digestive tract. So even though we remove the colon and rectum, if it is Crohn's, the inflammation could return elsewhere later on."

That was probably my biggest fear of all. What if I went through with the surgery, had my colon and rectum removed, and that still didn't put me into remission because the disease just came back somewhere else? This was the worst-case scenario. But at least I would not be shitting my pants anymore, because I would have the ostomy bag. That was where I was drawing the line for success at this point: Can you make it so I no longer shit my pants?

"I don't expect you to make a decision today," Dr. Stevens said off of the stunned looks on both my and my dad's faces. "Think about it. Talk it over with your family. Talk some more with Dr. Calvin. Today is only about presenting you with as much information as possible."

"I understand," I said. "I do have one more question. I'm thinking of everything I did to get ready for this appointment. And then, it, well... got rescheduled to today. Because of an emergency."

Dr. Stevens nodded. "Yes," he said.

"And I understand that things like that happen, of course," I added quickly. "But I'm just worried that... I don't know..." I fumbled for words, not sure how to express the concern that I had, but the look on Dr. Stevens's face indicated he knew what I was about to ask. "I would really hate for that to happen again. Does that happen often? Like, if I did elect to do this surgery, is there any chance it would end up getting canceled for an emergency?"

"No," Dr. Stevens said confidently. Then, after a moment, he added, "Your surgery would *be* the emergency."

Chapter Twenty-Nine

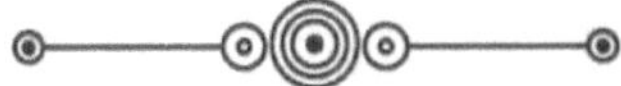

At my next acupuncture session with Teagan, I told her I was considering the ileostomy surgery.

"Please don't do that," she said, seeming alarmed. "Give me a little more time to see what I can do for you. I would hate to have you do that if we can get you better holistically."

I understood how extreme this surgery must seem to anyone else. But I was quickly starting to feel like it was the only option I had left. I had given so many other things a chance at this point, and I was still a mess. I wished that I knew what to do. I appreciated that Teagan wanted more time to try to get me better with herbs and acupuncture. I just didn't know how much time I had left to give.

On November 30, I heard back about the job application I had put in at the payroll company. They wanted me to come in for an interview. I went in and worked my usual early-morning shift at 13 WHAM that day, then went home, put on a suit and tie, and drove out for my interview. On the way, I popped an Imodium. I couldn't risk having to run out of the interview to use the bathroom.

The company had multiple locations in Rochester. I was not interviewing at the same building that my dad worked at. I walked up to the front desk and told the receptionist I was there for an interview. I was a little bit early, so I asked if I could use the restroom before we got started. That way I could get out anything that was "on deck" before the interview began while I waited for the Imodium to stop everything else in its tracks.

The interview was with three managers in a small conference room. It was a little intimidating at first—it felt like three against one! But everyone was pleasant and professional. The interview really felt more like a conversation.

This is going to sound counterintuitive, but there is a strange sort of calm that can come with being constantly stressed. I remember one time when I was filling in as director of the eleven p.m. news at 13 WHAM and we were having to make a bunch of changes to the next segment while we were in a commercial break. Someone said to me, "You are always so calm; it's like you never get stressed out."

How ironic was that comment? It's like a duck on the water. Everyone sees the duck quietly gliding along. What they can't see is his little duck feet kicking like crazy under the surface. For me, it was the fact that I was constantly trying to keep my Crohn's under control. If I could manage that, everything else seemed easy, like it was inconsequential by comparison.

For that reason, I felt confident and comfortable in the interview. In my mind, if I didn't shit my pants in front of everyone in the conference room, then anything else that happened was a resounding success. The managers presented me with a series of situational questions. What would you do if you had multiple high-priority tasks at the same time? How would you handle an upset customer? Can you tell me about a time when you were up against a tight deadline and how you handled it?

I was honest and open, but I also felt like I was playing a character. I was pretending to be the version of me that I wanted to be. I wasn't lying about anything; all of the answers I gave were true and based on experiences I'd had in my previous jobs. I even managed to make everyone laugh a couple of times. In fact, I was downright charming. But in a way, I felt like I was acting. I was playing the role of a Russ Dimino who didn't have Crohn's disease, a fictional version of myself who had my shit together (no pun intended). I was letting them see the duck on top of the water. I left feeling like I had nailed the interview.

Less than a week later, I heard back from them. They were offering me the job! My first day would be Monday, December 28. This job was going to pay enough that I could quit 13 WHAM and Sam's Club and still be making more money than those two jobs combined. And better still, I had been scheduled to work Christmas Eve and Christmas Day at 13 WHAM. I got the offer in time to be able to put in my two-weeks' notice and be out of there by December 23! It truly was a Christmas miracle.

When I gave my notice at 13 WHAM, I was hoping they would've tried to keep me. Instead, the response I got was something to the effect of, "This is what always happens!" I couldn't help but think that maybe it was because they always kept people as part-timers so they didn't get any benefits. They did express that they were sorry to see me go, that they appreciated all of my hard work, and that I would be missed. I had gone in wondering what I would do if they had tried to counteroffer. What if they had offered to make me full time and give me regular hours and a raise so that I would stay? I guess I didn't need to worry about that. But they probably could have kept me there if they tried.

My coworkers were sad to hear about my imminent departure. They invited me and Amanda out for a farewell dinner at Buffalo Wild Wings. There was a pretty large turnout of producers, directors, my fellow production crewmembers, and even some of the anchors who all came out to wish me well in my next endeavor. It was Amanda's first time meeting many of them. There was a huge spread of various appetizers and finger foods, none of which I was comfortable eating, but of course I didn't want anyone to know that. Amanda and I "shared" a plate of food. I expertly moved things around like an actor on a TV show, never actually taking a bite. At end of the dinner, legendary news anchor Don Alhart read a poem he had written about me. This was something he often did when a longtime member of the 13 WHAM staff left or retired; I was the first part-time employee he had ever done that for. Then they presented me with a giant, oversized card made on a piece of posterboard. A coworker had drawn a picture of me as Superman on the front of the card, flying away from the 13 WHAM building! Everyone at the station had signed it.

I was speechless. I truly hadn't known I meant that much to everyone. I had a pang of regret thinking about how much more I could have enjoyed my time there if I had been healthy. My disease had kept me from truly having fun at a job that I really did like a lot. I wished I could've somehow started over and done it all again with a clean bill of health. Instead, I would have to settle for putting on my cape and flying off into the sunset.

My new job was very different from anywhere I had worked before. I had my own cubicle, which somehow seemed exciting. A desk where there was a nameplate with my name on it felt reassuring to someone who had juggled part-time jobs with ever-changing hours for so long. It felt like I had a little piece of property. It was proof that yes, they really did want me there.

The implementation coordinator role involved working with clients over the phone and via webinar to configure and utilize their time and attendance product—a website that allowed them to track their employees' hours worked, schedules, time-off requests, etcetera. Then they would have all of that data accessible and importable when they ran payroll.

The clients I worked with had already signed up for the service, so it's not like I was having to cold-call or sell anyone on anything. They would be expecting my call, and I would be assisting them with learning to use a product that they had already said that they wanted. It was a nice change of pace, and a chance for me to flex some different muscles than I had been using previously.

Of course, my Crohn's symptoms required me to adapt my old song and dance to a new environment. I was still slipping away multiple times per day to use the restroom. In the early days of my new role, this meant literally getting up and walking out of training class or stepping away from a team member's desk in the midst of shadowing a call with them. Fortunately, no one asked me what I was doing or where I was going. I just tried to be fast and discreet and return to where I was supposed to be as quickly as I could.

One day we were all in the conference room for a team meeting, and one of my colleagues did raise the subject.

"Hey," Ellie, one of the other new hires I was in training with, said to me in front of everyone. "I stopped by your desk a few times looking for you. You're never there!"

My manager, who was leading the meeting, raised an eyebrow and leaned back in his chair.

"Hmm, that is weird," I said. "We must keep just missing each other." The answer made no sense. She had been looking for me, I had not been looking for her. But I said it so casually and with such confidence it seemed to settle the matter somehow. I had gotten really good at acting like things were normal. It was like I had a secret identity. Except instead of running off to a phone booth and ripping open my shirt, I was running off to the bathroom and dropping my pants.

The new job also came with new health insurance. The first time I tried to refill my Cimzia, there was an issue. I had been getting the Cimzia through CuraScript, a distributor that delivers certain types of prescriptions like biologics and infusible mediations directly to your home.

To be honest, I don't remember the details of whether my new insurance provider wouldn't work with CuraScript or CuraScript didn't accept my new insurance; I don't recall who had a problem with whom. All I knew was that now that I was on this new insurance, I was not going to be able to get the Cimzia delivered directly to me via CuraScript anymore.

I ended up saying screw it and just not refilling it. I don't recommend quitting a biologic agent, or any medication really, without talking to your doctor first. At this point I was just over it. I wasn't about to fight for the ability to keep sticking a syringe into my tummy every two weeks, full of something that did not even seem to be helping me. I was done.

Early into the new job, management asked a bunch of us to come in on a Saturday for some additional training that we hadn't been able to fit in during the week. They assured us that coming in on the weekend was not something that would usually be expected of us. It was a chance to earn some overtime, so I didn't mind much. But the invitation to this weekend work session included four little words that most people would be excited by, though they struck fear into my heart: "Lunch will be provided."

When I walked into the breakroom at lunchtime that day, there were a plethora of submarine sandwich trays on a table in the middle of the room. I craned my neck to see around the line of eager coworkers waiting to grab their grub. All of the sub rolls had seeds on them, and it looked like they were all piled high with lettuce, tomatoes, and various other fixings.

Now, I did occasionally eat subs, but I always got plain bread (no seeds) and definitely no lettuce. The leafy greens were just too hard for me to digest. If I wanted to partake in the subs, I'd have to take off all of the lettuce, and I'd probably try to pluck off most or all of the seeds on the roll as well. If I was in the comfort of my own home, I'd attempt it. But to sit in the breakroom surrounded by my new colleagues and start picking apart my meal like a finicky five-year-old? I couldn't do it.

I ducked back out of the breakroom before anyone noticed me. I went into the bathroom and into a stall and shut the door.

I thought for a minute about running out to get something else to eat. I didn't know the area very well yet though, so I wasn't sure what was around. And I was afraid someone might see me leaving and ask why I was going out for lunch when there was free food in the breakroom. I decided I would just hide until lunch was over.

While everyone else was enjoying lunch, I sat in the bathroom waiting out the clock. (The irony of the bathroom being my safe haven here was not lost on me.) As I waited, I could not help but think about how I was allowing the vicious cycle to continue. I wasn't just missing out on food. I was missing out on all my new coworkers getting to know each other. I was going to be the odd man out again. The quiet guy who never socialized with anyone. All so I could protect my crappy secret.

Needless to say, I almost always did my own thing when it came to lunch at work. One day I clocked out and decided to make a run to Wegmans. I was planning on getting a plain bagel. An untoasted, unbuttered hunk of bread to nibble on had become something that sounded good to me. At least it was something my volatile tummy could handle.

My lunch break was an hour long. The drive from the office to Wegmans was about ten, maybe fifteen minutes. So if I planned on half an hour of driving time round trip, that would give me half an hour to get my bagel and hopefully just sit quietly in my car and eat it in peace. That sounded nice.

I got to Wegmans and walked across the parking lot toward the entrance. It was especially cold that day, with lots of snow on the ground. The cold made my insides tingle and clench up. I knew it was triggering an episode for me and that I'd have to get to the bathroom ASAP. I picked up my pace and did my classic tight-legged jog into the store.

I quickly shuffled my way into the men's room. To my horror, it was a small restroom with a couple of urinals and one stall, which was occupied. Oh no. I could also tell by the lack of any sound or movement in the stall that the guy inside was not finishing up. He was parked in place and not going anywhere anytime soon.

I knew this Wegmans pretty well. There was another restroom on the second floor, above the café area. I was pushing my luck, but I was going to have to try to make it up the stairs to the other bathroom.

Again doing a clenched-up sprint-waddle, I made it to the stairs and ascended them as quickly as I could, just trying to keep everything in. I felt like a time bomb that was at the 0:01 mark, just about to tick that final tock.

I made it to the upstairs bathroom and threw open the door only to find that it also only had one stall. And it was also occupied.

There were two public men's room stalls in this whole building, and both of them were in use.

I walked back out in the hallway outside the men's room. No one else was around. I quietly, sadly soiled myself.

I hated this. I fucking hated it. The sharp stinging sensation in my abdomen. The dirty, uncomfortable feeling of the excrement forming in my diaper and sticking to my skin. The shame and embarrassment I felt even though no one knew what was happening. And at the same time, the numbness that came with the fact that this was just my life now. That this was not even an uncommon occurrence for me. And how unfair that was.

I waited and waited for the guy to come out of this upstairs bathroom. Many long minutes went by with me just standing there, waiting, trying to stay composed in my own filth. The guy was taking his sweet time. I found myself getting so angry that he had the pleasure of sitting on a toilet to defecate while I was standing outside in the hallway being denied that simple privilege. I hated him, and I hated the guy who was using the downstairs stall.

Finally I got tired of standing around waiting. With a diaper full of my own feces, I shambled my way downstairs to the first restroom to see if it was free yet. I found that yes, that stall was finally vacant. At least now I had some privacy for the unpleasant undertaking of changing myself. I went in the stall, took off my pants, removed my diaper and put it into one of the plastic bags I always carried with me, wiped myself, put on a new diaper, and put my pants back on.

Even as routine as this process had become, I always had to detach myself from it. I was going through the motions physically, but mentally I had to shut down. It's like I was a robot performing a task I had been programmed to do. I could not think about the reality of what I was doing. I couldn't allow myself to be present in the process of changing my shit-filled diaper in a Wegmans bathroom stall on my lunch break from work.

When all this was said and done, I had less than fifteen minutes left in my lunch break. That was not going to be enough time to go pick out a bagel, stand in the checkout line to pay for it, get back to my car, and drive back to work before I needed to clock back in.

I hustled back to my car without getting anything to eat.

As it was, I was still late punching back in.

I had spent my entire lunch driving to a store, soiling myself, changing my diaper, and driving back to work.

I could not keep living like this.

I just fucking couldn't.

That was the day, that was the moment, that I made the decision.

I was going to get the surgery.

Now that I had made the decision to definitely move ahead with the surgery, there was someone I wanted to tell in person. Teagan had tried so hard to help me get better. She had really seemed like she was trying to save me from needing the surgery. I was worried she would be disappointed or upset when she found out.

One day after work, I stopped by her office. She was in with a patient, so I waited around for a few minutes. Eventually she popped out of one of the rooms. She was surprised to see me.

"Hey! Do you have a minute?" I asked.

"Hey! Of course. What's up? Is everything okay?"

"Yeah, everything's fine. I just wanted to talk to you. I wanted to tell you about something that happened."

I launched into the story about the incident at Wegmans. About going there to try to get a quick bite to eat on my lunch break. About having an accident because the stall was in use. About the whole ordeal taking so long that I didn't even have time to get the bagel I was planning to get.

"And then I ended up being late getting back to work," I said.

"And they fired you?!" she exclaimed.

"What? No, no, they didn't fire me," I said. "Actually, they didn't even say anything about me being late. I'm not sure anyone even noticed." I thought it was funny that that's where she thought the story was going. I guess the situation could have been worse after all. "I just… I just can't do it anymore. This incident put me over the edge. I can't keep living like this. I'm going to get the surgery. I just wanted you to know. You've tried harder than anyone to help me, and I know you were really hoping you could help me avoid having that done. I just can't keep waiting and I just wanted to tell you in person."

She looked like she was going to cry. She nodded, then gave me a long hug.

"I understand," she said quietly. She sighed. "If only you could have come to me sooner. Maybe if we had started acupuncture earlier, I could've helped you."

"You did help me," I said. "You really did. I couldn't have made it this far without you."

It was a very emotional moment. I knew she couldn't help but feel like she had failed me somehow. And I couldn't help feeling like I was letting her down by choosing to get the surgery. And neither of us wanted the other to feel that way. The whole situation just sucked.

Chapter Thirty

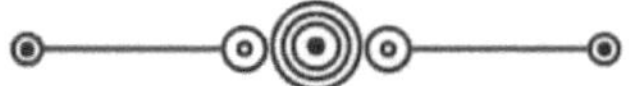

At my next appointment with Dr. Calvin, I told him that I had decided that I wanted to have the surgery. However, I wasn't ready to schedule it right away. I had been looking into my benefits at the new job, and I wouldn't qualify for short-term disability or sick pay until I had been there ninety days, and that wouldn't be until the end of March.

"There was something I was wondering if we could try in the meantime," I said. "I was wondering about low-dose naltrexone."

Dr. Calvin crossed his arms and leaned back in his chair. "Look, I'll be honest," he said. "I have had some patients who had success going into remission with LDN. But they all had much milder cases than you do. With everything else that you've already tried, and how severe your symptoms are, I don't think that LDN is going to be strong enough to do the trick for you, Russ, I really don't."

"It's just that, to me, the surgery really feels like a last resort," I said. "I want to feel like I've tried absolutely everything else before going into it, like I didn't leave any other stone unturned. As long as we have a couple of months, can we at least give it a shot?"

Dr. Calvin sighed. "All right," he said. "You make a good argument. We can give it a try if you want to. You can't get it filled just anywhere, though. You need to go to a compounding pharmacy, because we are filling it at a dose that's lower than normal due to it being an off-label prescription in this case. Do you know where the Twelve Corners Apothecary is?"

"No," I said.

"It's in the Twelve Corners, man!" he said, laughing.

The Twelve Corners was an area in Brighton where Monroe Avenue, South Winton, and Elmwood Avenue all crossed over to form a kind of triangular intersection with a shopping center right in the middle. It actually was not far from where I was working now. He wrote the prescription out for me and told me I needed to take it there.

"By the way, if you do proceed with the surgery, you'll need to stop taking the LDN forty-eight hours before the surgery, since it blocks the effects of narcotics," Dr. Calvin continued. "And as long as we have a little time, there is one other thing I would like to do. I think I mentioned the Prometheus test before. It's a blood test that can help us differentiate whether you actually have Crohn's disease or ulcerative colitis. That will be helpful for us to know going into the surgery. Dr. Stevens probably explained why?"

"Yes," I said. "If it's colitis, the surgery is a cure. If it's Crohn's… it's… well, if it's Crohn's then it's not."

"Correct," Dr. Calvin said. "It's time to know which one we are dealing with."

I would say you're not going to believe this, dear reader, but if you've made it this far into the story, you probably will. The Prometheus test was inconclusive.

Dr. Calvin gave me a call to break the news.

"The Prometheus blood test can accurately detect Crohn's disease in about 77% of patients, and colitis in slightly less than that. You apparently fall into the minority in which it doesn't detect either one," he said. "This isn't unheard of. I had a patient once who had Crohn's disease so bad that he had to essentially have emergency surgery because of it, and yet the blood test showed no inflammatory bowel disease."

"Dr. Calvin, is it at all possible that I don't have Crohn's or colitis, but something else entirely?" I asked. "I haven't responded to any of the usual treatments, and now the blood test doesn't show either disease. Is there any chance we are dealing with something else?"

"I expected you to ask that," Dr. Calvin said. "No, the real gold standard is the biopsy, not the blood test. The biopsies from your last colonoscopy are diagnostic of inflammatory bowel disease, and the endoscopic appearance was diagnostic of that as well. That's the question I expected you to ask, though. You didn't let me down!"

I was more confused than ever now. Why didn't anything about my case fit neatly into any boxes? It made me start to wonder about the labels that we put on things when we get sick. Does everything always fall into a category that we as humans have seen before and given a name to? Do we always get sick in the same way that someone else before us has already gotten sick? Couldn't something go wrong with your body without it "being" something?

I went and got the LDN filled at the Twelve Corners Apothecary. If not for the sign out front telling you that it was a business, the place just looked like it was somebody's house. Inside it was very quaint and had an old-school, rustic feel to it, with row upon row of wooden cabinets containing all kinds of bottles of different shapes and sizes.

A compounding pharmacy is able to customize medications from how they are commercially available; in the case of LDN, altering it to a lower dose than patients who take it to treat narcotic addictions. They can also alter prescriptions to remove preservatives or inactive ingredients that the patient might be allergic to. I thought for a moment about how I'd switched temporarily from taking prednisone in pill form to liquid form when Dr. Griswold said I had a lactose intolerance. If I had known about this place back then, maybe they could have customized something for me.

I got my LDN prescription filled. It was a very strange feeling, because it occurred to me that this was the last thing that I was going to try. It was either going to work, or I was going to have surgery. Either way, there would not be anything else after this one. Somehow getting it filled at such a unique place felt appropriate. Now I could really and truly say I had tried everything.

Chapter Thirty-One

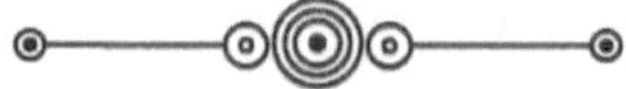

One weekend in mid-February 2010, I got hit with a bad stomach bug. I was vomiting and could not keep anything down.

I was lying in bed. Amanda brought me a glass of water and a Gatorade.

"You have to be sure to stay hydrated," she said. "Take small sips, but make sure you keep drinking."

I took a small sip of the Gatorade. Within a minute or two, I was vomiting again.

I tried the water. Again, the smallest sip I could muster. Once again, vomiting. Introducing anything to my system was forcing it into "eject" mode before it could even hit my stomach.

Amanda would check on me every so often and ask why I hadn't had any of my water or Gatorade. I'd tell her my stomach wasn't ready for it yet, to give me more time. I would assure her I was working on it, that I just needed to go really slow. She would make me promise to drink some more before she came back again, and I'd tell her that I would. But again, every time I took even a tiny sip, I ended up vomiting. Eventually I just stopped trying. It didn't make sense to keep trying to drink anything if it was just going to induce vomiting each time.

On Monday, I called in sick to work. I hated calling in sick so soon—I had only been working there for a little over a month. I told my boss that I had a stomach bug and couldn't make it in. He did not seem upset; he told me just to rest up and feel better.

Amanda urged me to try to take a shower, since it had been a couple of days. She said it might perk me up, but I suspect it was also because I was getting a bit ripe.

I got in the shower, but I was so woozy I could barely stay standing. I was so lightheaded, I felt like I might fall. As long as I was in there, I figured I should at least shampoo my hair. I quickly lathered up my hair and immediately rinsed it back out. The whole time, I was just trying to stay standing and get done as fast as I possibly could.

As soon as I got the shampoo out of my hair, I turned the shower off. My body felt cold and shivery; I had not even stayed in long enough to adjust to the temperature. As I started drying off, I was seeing little pops of light through a dingy haze.

I stumbled back to the bedroom and collapsed onto the bed, naked and still damp. I just needed to lie down. The effort of standing up long enough to take a shower was too much. I was too weak. I don't know if I had even been in the shower for a full minute. The room was spinning as I looked up at the ceiling. This was awful. I just wanted it to stop.

Before Amanda left for work, she set me up on the couch in the living room with a blanket, a pillow, and more Gatorade, which I still was not drinking. I think she thought a change of scenery from the bedroom would do me some good, even if I was still just lying down and resting.

"Do you want me to put something on the TV for you before I leave?" she asked.

"No." I laughed, as if that was absurd. "I can't even see the TV with all these…"

I stopped mid-sentence. What had I been about to say? I was going to say I can't see the TV with all these buildings in the way. But that didn't make sense. Why was I going to say that? For some reason I had thought, just for a moment, that I was on a rooftop overlooking a city skyline, and there were so many buildings blocking my field of view that I couldn't see the TV.

But I was lying on the couch. How could I have been seeing buildings? Why was I so sure that was what I had been about to say, and how could I really finish that sentence? I waved my hand in the air, trying to grasp for the right words. "You know," I finally said. "You know what I mean, right?"

Amanda just looked confused. She looked at the coffee table next to me. "Is your Gatorade blocking your view of the TV?" she asked.

"No," I said, shaking my head, frustrated but also kind of embarrassed. I kind of knew I wasn't making sense, but I also knew there was something I had really intended to say that had seemed logical when I started to say it. "You know what I mean,"

I said again. "I just can't think of the word. There's too many... you know. In the way."

I was delirious and starting to hallucinate. I was so dehydrated that my mind was not functioning correctly. But I did not understand this at the time.

Amanda left for work, and I spent the day fading in and out of consciousness on the couch. I did not drink any of the Gatorade, convinced it would only send me into another vomiting fit and thinking that would just be counterproductive. I did still have to bolt up the stairs to the bathroom to evacuate my bowels every so often.

Sprinting to the bathroom when I could hardly stand up without feeling dizzy was tantamount to torture. I would be lying on the couch, trying to sleep, and I'd feel my stomach tightening up and that familiar pressure winding its way through my guts. I would know I was going to have to run to the bathroom, but I'd try to delay it. I would be in denial for a bit, hoping maybe I was wrong and I would not have to go and I could just keep lying there.

But eventually it would prove inevitable. In a burst of adrenaline, I would make the herculean effort to run up the stairs fast enough to make it to the toilet before the dizziness had time to take hold of me. It did not really work. One time I was so woozy that I misjudged where the toilet was and fell on the floor. My vision was an overlay of gray and flashes of light.

It wasn't fair. All I wanted to do was rest.

When Amanda got home, I was back in bed, having abandoned the couch since the bedroom was closer to the bathroom.

"Did you drink any of your Gatorade?" she asked me. "I still see a full bottle down there."

"No," I said.

"Why not? Russ, you need to be drinking a lot of fluids."

"Every time I drink anything, I throw up."

Amanda looked at me. I was pale and my eyes were glassy and unfocused. She looked genuinely scared.

"When was the last time you drank anything and it actually stayed down?"

I honestly had no idea how much time had passed. "What day is it?" I asked.

"Are you telling me you have not kept any liquids down for three days now?" she asked.

"I don't know," I said. I really could not remember.

"Russ, I think we should get you to the doctor," Amanda said.

I just grunted. What was the doctor going to do? I had a stomach bug. A virus. They don't give you anything for that. You just need to rest and let it run its course. This was taking a long time to run its course, but eventually I would get through it and feel better. I just needed to wait it out. There was no point in going to the doctor.

"Russ," Amanda said. "You have Crohn's. Your immune system is probably having a hard time kicking this. And with the medicines you're on, they always say to take any infections very seriously, right?"

"Hm."

"The fact that you haven't been able to keep anything down at all for days is worrying me. I would really like you to go to the doctor."

I just kept lying there.

"I'm going to call and make you an appointment. Okay?"

"Mm," I said.

Amanda left the room and called the doctor's office. We were able to get an appointment at my primary care doctor's office that afternoon with one of the nurse practitioners.

I managed to put some clothes on—sweatpants and a long-sleeve T-shirt. Even just walking out to the car took all my concentration and focus; it was a chore just to put one foot in front of the other, walk out the door, and get into the car. I was weak and lightheaded, and I had a complete lack of energy.

Just riding to the doctor's office was hard. To be clear, I did not have to do anything but sit there, and the doctor's office was maybe a ten-minute drive from our house. But just sitting there in the car, in the daylight, watching the road go by out the window, I felt so… exposed. I was out in the harsh world, away from my couch and my bed and my bathroom. I had to "hold it together" now, and even just sitting in the passenger seat of the car with my wife at the wheel felt like I was using up energy I didn't have. I felt like Senator Kelly right before he devolves into a puddle of water in the first *X-Men* movie.

When we got to the doctor's office, I was taken in to see a physician assistant named Cara. She asked me about my symptoms, how long they had been going on, and when the last time was that I had been able to keep any food or water down. I answered the questions in short one- or two-word fragments, trying to conserve the energy it took even to talk. Amanda filled in some gaps for me. Amanda and Cara were both looking at me like they were looking at a ghost. It's frightening how close it was to that being accurate.

Suddenly I felt another huge wave of nausea bubbling up from the depths of my stomach.

"I need to throw up," I said.

Cara looked around the exam room, wide-eyed. She grabbed a small pink plastic basin and thrust it into my hands. I heaved forward and retched, somehow coming up with more contents from my starved stomach and upchucking them into the basin. I don't know what I could have been throwing up at that point besides pure bile.

I blinked my watery eyes again and again, not able to bring myself to look at Amanda or Cara.

"I'm sorry," I choked out between vomits.

"You don't need to be sorry," Cara said, her voice gentle but concerned.

"I know… but… I'm still sorry," I said as I kept retching up liquid. I felt ashamed.

I clung to the pink basin like a security blanket long after I was done puking.

"Mr. Dimino, I need you to go to the emergency room," Cara said. "They can get you an IV to get some fluids in you and give you something to stop the vomiting. I can call an ambulance for you to take you there."

"No," I said, shaking my head. "Don't need an ambulance. We can just drive there."

There was a long pause.

"Is there a reason you don't want to take an ambulance?" she asked.

There were a couple of reasons going through my mind. One was that ambulances were expensive. I had so many bills piled up already, I didn't need one more. The second thing was that even at this point, I felt like everyone was making too big of a fuss over me, that this was not the big deal everyone was acting like. If I needed to go the hospital to get an IV, that's fine, but Amanda could just drive me there.

"It just seems…" I tried to figure out how to condense my thoughts into as few words as possible. "…unnecessary," I finally settled on.

"With all due respect, Mr. Dimino, I think it is necessary," Cara said. There was something more than just concern in her voice. It was like she was deliberately trying to keep her tone even to keep from alarming me or Amanda. "They will get you in much faster if you go by ambulance. They can start the admission process while you are en route. It will take a lot longer if you go in on your own."

This was the first time the seriousness of this really started to sink in. Not only was I being told I needed to go to the hospital, but I needed to get there as quickly as possible.

"Okay," I relented. "Okay. Ambulance is okay."

Cara stepped out of the room to go call the ambulance. Amanda and I just looked at each other. My eyes were still watery from my latest vomiting episode. I still felt embarrassed from puking in front of them.

"I think taking the ambulance is the right decision, Russ," she said.

"Okay," I said back. It was all I could say. I was beyond exhausted. I just wanted to rest.

Before long, they put me in a wheelchair and took me out a back door of the doctor's office. Someone took my pink puke bucket to wash it out, which made me anxious. The ambulance was waiting outside, and Cara was talking to one of the EMTs. It was reassuring to know I was going right from her care to the ambulance and would not have to tell someone what was going on all over again.

Amanda knelt down beside me and said she was going to follow along in the car right behind the ambulance, and that she would call my parents and let them know what was going on. "I wish I could ride in the ambulance with you," she said. I knew she did not want to leave my side. But she was also very practical and knew it did not make sense to leave our car at the doctor's office. "I'll be right behind you, and I'll see you as soon as we get there, okay?"

The EMTs loaded me into the ambulance, and we were on our way.

Fortunately, they gave me back my pink bucket because I threw up again in the ambulance. My eyes were plastered shut with sweat and tears from the strain of puking. I just kept thinking I wanted this to be over.

When we got to Rochester General Hospital, the admission process was quick. After they took me out of the ambulance and I was lying on the stretcher in a small admissions area, one of the EMTs who brought me there was talking to a nurse who was entering notes on a laptop computer. As they were doing that, I tried to imagine what it would have been like if Amanda drove me to the hospital and we'd had to just walk in and sit in the waiting room. Heck, we would probably still be sitting in traffic.

They wheeled me over to a small curtained-off room in the ER to get me going on an IV. Amanda and my parents came back to see me shortly after that; my parents had hopped right in the car after getting the call from Amanda. Even now, I still had a kind of embarrassed feeling like everyone was making too much fuss over me. That feeling was still outweighing any feelings of being afraid.

The nurse who got me hooked up to the IV also brought me some blankets. He had noticed I was shivering. My mom would later remark that the nurse was cracking jokes left and right to try to get me to laugh or smile and that I had not even reacted to any of it. That's when she became really concerned, when she noticed I had no response whatsoever to the one thing that usually got me through anything: humor.

They got me admitted to a room for the night with the plan of just keeping me on the IV to try to get me hydrated again. I spent the night just lying in a bed getting fluids dripped into my veins.

The next day, a doctor came in to speak with me. He told me that I was very fortunate to have come to the hospital when I did, and that I had been on the verge of kidney failure. The creatinine level—a waste product that is normally filtered out by your kidneys—for an adult male should be around 0.6 to 1.2 mg/dL. When I got to the hospital, mine was close to 9 mg/dL. This indicated that my kidneys were shutting down.

The doctor told me that if I had waited another day to get medical attention, I probably would have died. This news hit me like a ton of bricks. I had really come that close to death's door? And the whole time I had been reluctant to even go to the doctor, thinking that there was nothing they would do for a virus.

I looked at Amanda. I had almost made her a widow after a little over a year of marriage. She could have been planning my funeral right now. Yet again, the words of Dr. Harvey hung over me like a storm cloud: *You will have a shorter life span.* I had almost punched my ticket at age twenty-seven.

It was a wake-up call to all of us. My family did not leave my side the whole time I was in the hospital. There was always someone—Amanda, my mom, or my dad—with me every day. My mom asked me if there was anything I wanted her to get from the house, like my laptop or anything like that. I said yes to the laptop, and then, reluctantly, asked if she could bring me my

Depends from the bedroom closet. That was a hard moment for me, to admit to my mother that her son was wearing adult diapers.

At this point, though, did it really make sense to keep anything a secret? She brought me my laptop and my Depends, and she even stopped at my favorite comic book store and bought me a stack of comics. The idea of my mom going into the comic store made me smile just as much as having the actual reading material.

By Friday my kidneys had finally returned to normal functionality, and I was discharged from the hospital. The minute we got home, Amanda went into the kitchen to start making me some chicken soup.

I thought back to all of the times I had been cautioned that I needed to take infections very seriously due to the immunosuppressant meds I was on. Even the fact that I couldn't kick those warts without laser treatments should have told me that my body was not able to heal itself the way a normal person's would.

I needed to get off these drugs. They were compromising my whole well-being at this point, and they weren't even suppressing my Crohn's. What good were they doing me? I was already sick enough, and the stuff that was supposed to be helping me only seemed to be doing even more damage.

My illness had quite literally become a matter of life and death.

Chapter Thirty-Two

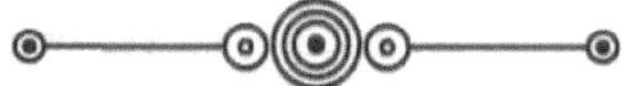

It was time to shit or get off the pot, if you'll pardon the very appropriate expression. The LDN, much as Dr. Calvin had predicted, was not even making a dent in my symptoms. I scheduled the total proctocolectomy with ileostomy surgery with Dr. Stevens for April 2010.

Now I had to let work know I was going to be taking some time off. I stopped by my manager's desk at work and asked if we could talk privately for a minute. He said sure, and we grabbed an empty conference room.

"What's on your mind?" he asked.

"Um, I'm not really sure how to start this conversation," I said. "Are you familiar with Crohn's disease?"

He held up a hand. "I'm going to stop you right there," he said. "You don't need to tell me anything about your health if you don't want to."

"I understand that," I said. I flashed back again to the hospital in Virginia where I had asked them to write a note for Walmart explaining why I was in the hospital, and they informed me I absolutely did not need to give that information. It always felt like such a balancing act to me. I felt like I wanted to "prove" to my employer that I really did need to be out of work, that I had a good reason, even though I knew that legally I wasn't required to do so.

At the same time, that clashed with my instinct to keep my illness private. In this case, though, I trusted my manager and didn't want him to be in the dark about what was going on. "I won't go into a ton of detail. But I do want you to at least have an idea of what's happening. The short version is, I have Crohn's, and my doctor is recommending surgery. I'll be out of work for probably four to six weeks." Before he could even respond, I added, "I'm sorry."

"Don't be sorry," he said, shaking his head. "Thank you for trusting me with that information. I want you to know that that will stay between you and me. As far as the rest of the team is concerned, if they ask me where you are, I'll just say that you needed to take some time off and that will be the end of the conversation. You need to do what you need to do."

"Thank you. I really appreciate that," I said.

"The only thing I do want to make sure you are aware of," he continued a little more reluctantly. "You've been here... what, three months?"

"Yes," I said. I knew it was three months because that was long enough for me to have sick time and be eligible for short-term disability.

"FMLA doesn't kick in until you've been here for a year," he said.

I had no idea that FMLA and short-term disability were two different things, or that I needed to wait longer for one than the other. "Essentially, FMLA protects your job while you're away. Without that, that's not something that's guaranteed. There's a chance that you could come back from your leave, and the company could basically say, hey, we don't need you anymore."

Crap. I did not know about this part of the equation at all. I had finally gotten a stable Monday-to-Friday full-time job with benefits. Going out for the surgery might be putting that at risk. I let this sink in for a minute. Could I put the surgery off for another nine months? No. I couldn't. I would have to take the chance that I might come out of this unemployed.

"I… don't think this surgery is something that can wait that long," I said.

"That's fine," he said, putting up a hand again. "That is 100% between you and your doctor. I want you to do what's best for you. I'm just letting you know. And Russ, your work so far has been great. If it's up to me, you will have a place on the team when you get back. And if something happens at the company level where they don't want to hold that spot for you, I would be willing to help you find something else here if it comes to that."

"Thank you," I said. That meant a lot to me. I had only been there a few months, so I was glad to know I had made that strong of an impression. I understood that he was not promising anything. But him saying that made me feel valued and put some of my fear at ease. And ultimately, if that still didn't work out, I could always find something else. What I couldn't do was keep putting off the surgery. I had sacrificed my quality of life for long enough.

Two days before the surgery, Amanda and I met with an ostomy nurse who would measure me for where my ileostomy would go and show me what the appliance would look like. I will never forget that first meeting with Mary. She was very matter-of-fact and didn't really show much warmth or empathy for the situation I was in. I don't think she meant to be cold—she was just so used to it that I don't think it really occurred to her what it must be like for someone who is brand new to the idea that they are going to be having this huge change in their life.

Mary showed us an ostomy bag. It was an opaque plastic pouch, measuring about ten inches long and maybe five or six inches wide, that attached right to your skin with an adhesive ring on the back of the bag. There was an opening at the bottom of the bag with a Velcro flap to keep it shut. You simply undid the flap to empty waste from the bag into the toilet, then sealed it back up.

Next, Mary took out a measuring tape and measured my waist and where my belt line was. Then, based on her measurements, she took out a magic marker and drew a spot on my stomach. She covered the spot with a piece of clear packing tape so it wouldn't wash off. That was it. That was the spot where my ostomy would be. Something so precise and permanent marked off with something so quick and crude.

As Amanda and I walked out to the car, I could feel the tape on my stomach crinkling and pulling with each step. I thought, *I can't wait until I can take this tape off.* Then it hit me. I would not be taking it off. The tape would stay on until my surgery to keep the marker from washing or rubbing off. It would come off my body when Dr. Stevens took it off to perform the surgery. When I woke up, I would have an ostomy bag there, which I would have for the rest of my life. There would never just be plain, unblemished skin in that spot ever again.

I freaked out. I threw my keys on the ground and didn't get into the car. I sat down on the pavement and burst into tears. I buried my face in my hands and sobbed so hard I was shaking. Years of holding back all of my pain and fear came flooding out. The dam had burst. Amanda sat down next to me, rubbing my back and telling me that it was okay.

"I don't know if this is the right thing to do," I said through my tears. "What if I'm making a mistake?"

There was no going back from this. They were going to remove my entire colon and rectum. Once it was done, it was done; it's not like I could change my mind later on. There was something else that scared me too. What if Amanda didn't find me attractive anymore? I was going to have a hole in my gut with a bag of excrement attached to it for the rest of my life. I was so worried that she would find me repulsive after this surgery. Honestly, I found the whole thing repulsive myself. If I found it disgusting, how could she not?

We sat on the ground outside the car for a long time, me crying and pouring my heart out with all the worries that I'd been keeping inside. Amanda listened and let me get it all out. She held my hand and leaned her head on my shoulder.

"I don't know what to do," I said. "I'm not sure that I want to do this."

"I know it's scary," Amanda said. "But can you really keep living the way that you are now?"

I shook my head. No. I couldn't. And that was what it came down to. I had tried everything else. This was what was left.

April 15, 2010, the day before the surgery. I had to "prep" one last time, just like I would have for a colonoscopy. It felt different this time. Mentally, at least. As I prepped for each colonoscopy, I always knew I was doing it so that they could go up into my guts, poke around up there, and maybe find some information or see something that helped them know what to do to make me better.

As I sat on the bowl evacuating my intestines there was always the thought of, *Man, I hope this is worth it. I hope they learn something this time. I hope this isn't all for nothing.* This time, I knew I was cleaning things out for the last time. I was emptying my colon so they could go in and cut the whole thing out.

As I sat on the toilet in our basement that night, feeling my guts contract and convulse, I thought, *Go ahead. Do your worst. This is your last chance to glue my ass to this seat and make me go through this. Tomorrow you're done. You're getting cut out of me and you can burn in hell.*

The Crohn's disease demon had possessed my bowels and held my life hostage for the past five years. Tomorrow that son of a bitch was going to get exorcised.

April 16. Surgery day. Rochester General Hospital, in the early morning. I was lying on the gurney in the hallway of the hospital, waiting to be wheeled into surgery. Amanda and my mom were standing next to me. The anesthesiologist came over and put a saline lock into my hand and hooked me up to the IV that would be used to put me under. He assured me that he would be monitoring me closely during the whole surgery and would keep me nice and knocked out. I was so tired I felt like I could sleep through anything even without the anesthesia.

The anesthesiologist stepped away for a bit while we waited for it to be time for my surgery. I watched people rushing up and down the hallway, and it felt like a time lapse. Everything was blurring by while I lay still, suspended, waiting for it to be my turn to be wheeled in. I was anxious but not afraid. If anything, I felt eager. I was ready to be on the other side of this.

Then I felt that familiar urge. I could not believe it. I needed to use the freaking bathroom.

"Hey," I said, hating that I even had to say this sentence yet again. "I have to use the bathroom one more time."

"Okay," my mom said. There was concern in her voice, but never any frustration or judgment. She went a few steps and peered down the hall. "It looks like there's a men's room at the end of this hallway," she said. She stayed calm even though I felt a little panicky. I was already hooked up to the IV. Was I even able to get off this gurney?

Amanda helped me untangle myself from the cords and the tubes. The IV pole was on wheels, so I could get up and walk with it. I got off the gurney and wheeled my IV down the hallway to the bathroom.

As I sat on the toilet, one last harsh burst of bile blowing out of my bowels, I gritted my teeth and shook my head at the absurdity of it. Of course I would have to go again. Of course I would need to use the bathroom as I'm waiting to have my colon cut out. My stupid Crohn's demon had to get in one last laugh.

"It's weird to think about," I said as I got back on the gurney a few minutes later and tried to get comfortable. "That's hopefully the last time I will ever have to do that."

My mom laughed as though she hadn't thought of it that way.

I could not think of anything else.

The anesthesiologist who had hooked me up to the IV came back over. "Hey," he said. "When the doctor comes over, ask him how he slept last night." He had a big smile on his face, like he was letting me in on a joke.

Doctor Stevens came over. He asked if I had any questions about the procedure.

"How'd you sleep last night, doc?" I asked.

The anesthesiologist covered his mouth and tried to hide the fact that he was laughing.

"Fine," Dr. Stevens said, stone serious. "I slept fine."

The anesthesiologist gave me a fist bump.

I gave Amanda my glasses to hold on to. She took my hand and squeezed it tight. "I'll see you in a bit," she said. She was trying to sound casual, but her voice broke a little, giving her away. I squeezed back.

"I love you," I said.

"I love you too," she said with a soft smile.

Then they wheeled me down the hallway to the operating room.

As they were getting everything set up, my new anesthesiologist friend pointed at something several feet away. "That's the laser they use for the operation," he said. Without my glasses, it just looked like a big blurry gray mass. For all I could see, it might as well have been the Doctor Octopus arms from *Spider-Man 2*, and Dr. Stevens was about to do the surgery with four mechanical tentacles. In fact, that was exactly what I was picturing. This was my last thought as the anesthesiologist started the drip into my bloodstream that would lull me into a cozy, comfortable sleep.

Several hours later, I woke up to the realization that I couldn't breathe.

I opened my eyes. Everything was still blurry without my glasses, but I was able to tell that I was in a recovery area now and not the operating room. I couldn't breathe and couldn't figure out why. I was still so groggy it was hard to focus. I tried to turn my head or sit up, but I couldn't; I was still so sedated that my body didn't respond to the faint signals my brain was lazily sending down its neurons with no real sense of urgency. My mind was a paradox of utter panic and total apathy.

I had to really focus and try to push the mental fog away. Like trying to wake up from a dream, I mustered up all the effort that I could and tried to jerk my head to the side. It took a tremendous effort, but I managed to overcome my daze long enough to turn my head. I coughed a couple of times, finding my breath again. I took deep breaths, reminding my lungs that they needed to work.

There was a steady beep-beep-beep of a monitor tracking my vital signs not far from my head. How long would I have been breathless before it registered my distress?

A few feet away, a nurse was at a workstation, typing on a laptop.

I tried to tell her I was awake. The words wouldn't come out. I was trying to talk, but the words were not finding their way from my brain to my mouth.

"M'awake," I finally managed to murmur. "M'awake," I said again, a bit louder.

"We can't move you anywhere until your anesthesia wears off," the nurse said curtly without looking away from her screen. I had worked so hard to get those words out for such a dismissive response.

"Just wanted someone to know," I said sadly. (Although it came out more like, "Juss winnid summon no.")

She looked at me. "Okay," she said, much gentler and more sympathetic this time. "Thank you for letting me know. Just try to rest and relax."

I wanted to tell her how I hadn't been able to breathe for a minute. How I'd had to use all my strength to move my head and to be able to cough. But there was no way I could have articulated all of that. And it didn't matter.

I closed my eyes. I thought about the fact that I must have the ostomy bag now. I wanted to look at it, or at least touch it. I couldn't. I was in so much of a daze, stuck in that twilight state between awake and asleep. I let the edges of the world soften again as the constant beeping of my own vital signs soothed me back into a state of unconsciousness.

Chapter Thirty-Three

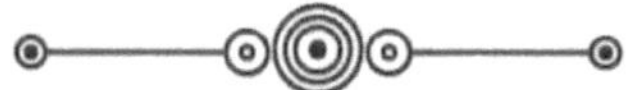

They moved me to a semi-private room in the hospital for my stay. "Semi-private," if you don't know, is a nice way of saying, "not private at all," because you are sharing a room with another patient and you are divided by a mere curtain. More on this in a bit.

My family came in to see me. We were told by Dr. Stevens that the surgery had gone very smoothly with no complications. This was amazing news. When I had a chance, I took a peek under my hospital gown to take a look at the ostomy bag. It was clear, unlike the opaque one Mary had shown me. I could see the bright-red stoma through it, and that freaked me out a little bit. I covered it back up. I'd have plenty of time to look at it, I figured. It wasn't like it was going anywhere.

Something else slowly dawned on me. Something felt different, but I couldn't quite put my finger on what it was. Then, like a lightbulb appearing over my head, I realized that the pain in my lower abdomen was gone. For years now, I'd had a constant dull, almost "itchy" kind of ache inside my abdomen, just below my belly button. Like I had a paper cut inside my guts. I had gotten so used to it that it felt normal to have that pain there. And now it was gone.

I felt like I had been holding my breath for five years. I finally exhaled.

For the first day in the hospital, I was on clear liquids only. That didn't really bother me, as I was so used to not eating anything as it was. Mostly I just felt tired, but for the first time in a long time, I could just rest without having to worry about rushing to the bathroom. That actually took a while to get used to. I was so used to having it in the back of my mind that I was going to need to run to the restroom that I had to retrain my brain not to worry about that anymore.

The ostomy bag was *really* going to take some getting used to. The first few times it needed to be emptied, a nurse came into the room and did it for me. They would take one of those pink puke basins, place it beside me on the bed, and then carefully open the bottom flap of my bag and squeeze the soupy brown sludge into the bin. I was so embarrassed and ashamed that I apologized to the nurse for having to do that.

Another thing that bothered me at first was that my ostomy was very noisy. Every few minutes, there would be a fart-like sound coming out of my stoma! How was I going to be able to keep this thing discreet if it was constantly passing gas? And unlike a "traditional" fart, there was no warning that it was coming, meaning there was no way to try to quietly conceal it. It just happened like a sudden trumpet blast. I was told that this would die down eventually, and that there was a lot of air that needed to pass through as a result of the surgery. I sure hoped so. The last thing I wanted was for people to do a double-take every time I farted out of the front of my stomach.

By the end of the first day, they wanted to have me try getting up and walking around. The sooner I was back on my feet, the sooner I could go home. Amanda and one of the nurses helped me up out of bed so I could try taking a little stroll. I was not prepared for how weak I felt. I hadn't taken more than a couple of steps before I felt dizzy and off-balance. I felt like the bottom half of my body couldn't support my top half.

"Help," I exclaimed. "I'm going to fall!" Amanda and the nurse grabbed my arms. They quickly guided me back to the bed.

"You did great," the nurse assured me. "You did really great."

"I did?" I asked. I had been out of bed and back into it in about ten seconds.

"Yes," she said. "You have to start somewhere. Your body has been through a tremendous ordeal, and you still got up and took a few steps. Tomorrow we'll see if you can do a few more."

I thought of a quote I had read once before, from Mary Anne Radmacher. "Courage does not always roar. Sometimes it is the quiet voice at the end of the day saying, 'I will try again tomorrow.'"

On day two, they wanted to start educating me a bit more on my ostomy. Amanda sat by my side so that she could learn about it too.

"You don't have to be here for this, you know," I said.

"Of course I do," she said. "What if you need help with it? I should know how it works too."

"I guess." I wasn't thrilled. I was still grossed out by the ostomy. I knew it was something I would have to learn to live with, and it was certainly better than the alternative of soiling my pants every day. Still, it was something I was reluctant to expose Amanda to. I was still afraid she would be turned off by it and not find me attractive anymore.

A nurse wheeled in a TV on a cart like you used to have brought into your classroom at school if the teacher was going to show a movie. "Watch this video, and let us know if you have any questions," she said. She pressed play on the VCR, and a video that looked like it had been made in the 1980s began. Had ostomy technology remained stagnant for thirty years? I couldn't tell whether the fact that these instructions had not required any updates since the Reagan administration was reassuring or cause for concern.

The nurse stepped out of the room. The video went over some basic ostomy care instructions. A lot of time was spent on how to empty the bag when it got full, as well as how to change it out for a new bag, which was something you generally had to do every few days. I was finding it very hard to pay attention to the video.

As I said, I was in a semi-private room, which meant I was sharing it with someone else. And it just so happened that right when Amanda and I were watching the ostomy care video was when my roommate had been discharged and was getting ready to go home. So as I'm watching the video, this guy's family is coming in and out of the room to help him gather up his stuff and move out. My side of the room was the side closest to the door, so every time someone came in or out they had to walk across my part of the room, right in between my bed and the TV.

At first it was distracting. Then it was embarrassing. Then it was downright mortifying. As the video was showing an animated depiction of emptying stool from the bag, strangers were walking through my room. This was something I was so self-conscious about that I barely wanted to share it with my wife. Now there were random people intruding on something I was having a hard enough time dealing with.

A woman walked past at one point—maybe my roommate's wife or girlfriend?—and gave me a sympathetic look. I don't know if she felt bad about the interruption or the fact that I had an ostomy, or both. I didn't care. I didn't want anyone else in here. I covered my face with my hands. I didn't want to look at anyone, and I didn't want to see the rest of the video. Amanda put her hand on my leg, unsure of what to do.

By the time my roommate and his family had finished moving out, the video was over. When the nurse came back in, I was fighting back tears.

"Hey, what's wrong?" she gasped.

"That... was really hard," I said, trying to compose myself. "This, um, this ostomy bag is something I'm struggling with—a lot. This is a big change and I'm pretty emotional about it. And having strangers walking in and out like that… um… it was just…" I started to tear up again. "That was just really tough."

"Oh my gosh. I am so, so sorry," she said. I could tell she really did feel bad. "I did not mean for that to happen. That should have been coordinated differently. I didn't realize that he was getting ready to leave right then."

"It's okay," I said. "It's not your fault." I couldn't even look at her, though. I was just staring down at the blankets. I felt humiliated.

"Hey," the nurse said after a moment. "I'll be right back, okay? I want to check on something." She stepped out of the room.

Amanda quietly held my hand as the two of us sat in silence.

After a couple of minutes, the nurse came back in. "Okay," she said. "There is no one else coming into this room today. You will have it to yourself for the rest of the day. And first thing tomorrow, we're going to move you to a private room. Would that make you feel better?"

I almost started crying again, out of happiness this time. "Yes." I nodded. "If you can make that happen, that would be so great."

"We will make it happen," she said.

After things had calmed down a bit, I had a question that I wanted to ask Amanda.

"If you had known that I was going to end up like this, would you have still wanted to be with me?" I asked.

"What do you mean?" she asked.

"Back before we started dating," I said. "If you had a crystal ball and it told you that I was going to get sick and that I was going to end up with an ostomy bag for the rest of my life, would you have still even wanted to date me?"

She considered the question very carefully. "Well, I don't know," she said after a moment. "Is that all that I would get to know?"

"I'm not sure what you mean," I said. I had kind of wanted her to immediately say yes, she would still want to be with me. But what she said next was so much better.

"When I'm looking into this crystal ball," she said, "is the fact that you would get sick and have an ostomy bag the only thing that I get to find out? Because if that's the only information it's giving me, then no, I probably wouldn't have dated you. But if it also told me what a kind and caring person you are, how smart you are, how funny you are, and what a great, loving, wonderful husband you would be… then yes. Of course I would have dated you, fallen in love with you, and married you, just like I did. I wouldn't change anything, Russ, unless there was a way that the crystal ball could have told me how to help you feel better sooner."

It was the absolute most perfect answer. It was what I needed to hear without knowing that I needed to hear it.

I tried walking again that evening. I was able to get all the way out of the room and a few steps into the hallway this time before I started feeling dizzy. By the day after that, Amanda and I were taking short walks up and down the hospital hallway. I knew that the sooner I could show them that I was ambulatory, the sooner they would consider letting me go home. I couldn't wait for a good night's sleep in my own bed.

While we were at the hospital, we got the news that Amanda's friend and coworker, Shannon, was at the very same hospital and had just given birth to a healthy baby girl, Madeline. Not sure of how far I could walk, Amanda snagged a wheelchair and covertly wheeled me over to the elevator.

We went up to the floor that had the maternity ward. You should've seen the look on the nurses' faces when they saw Amanda wheeling me, in my hospital gown, no doubt looking disheveled with bed-head and several days' worth of stubble, toward the nursery. For all they knew, she was bringing someone with an infectious disease toward the newborns. They went into panic mode, flagging us down and telling us we were in the wrong place.

Some lengthy explanations and apologies later, we were given permission to go in and visit. I hadn't seen a baby in a long time. Amanda cradled the sweet infant in her arms and talked gently to her. She looked very natural. I couldn't help but think, if my illness was finally under control, could a baby be in the future for me and Amanda too?

"Do you want to hold her, Russ?" Shannon asked me, startling me out of my thoughts.

"Oh, no, that's okay, I don't think I should," I replied. I was getting my strength back each day, but I was still unsteady on my feet and got tired quickly. I didn't think me holding a newborn was a good idea. It was still amazing to see her, though—those tiny hands, those little feet. Everything perfect, just miniaturized. A new life beginning, just as, in many ways, mine was beginning again as well.

As time went on, we were able to expand my diet. Clear liquids gave way to "full liquids"—soup, Jell-O, ice cream!—and then to solid foods. They gave me a little packet of graham crackers to eat, and I thought I had died and gone to heaven. Being able to eat something, even something as simple as a graham cracker, and not worry about having to run to the bathroom afterward for the first time in years, felt so liberating.

My dad was with me in the room when I ate the graham crackers, and he saw how happy I was.

"I'm going to go find you some more," he said.

"What?" I said. "You can't just go take them!"

"Sure I can!"

My dad casually walked around the hallway until he found the little pantry-like room where they kept the Jell-O cups, saltines, and other assorted snacks. He came back with a huge stack of graham crackers and a bunch of little cups of fruit juice. I laughed harder than I had in a long time.

Even better news was still to come. Dr. Calvin stopped by to see me and let me know that the pathology report from my colon—yes, they ran tests on my colon after removing it— indicated the findings were more consistent with ulcerative colitis than Crohn's disease.

This was the absolute best news I could have hoped for. Colitis meant that the disease was never going to come back. I didn't have to stay on medication at all anymore.

Colitis meant I was cured.

Chapter Thirty-Four

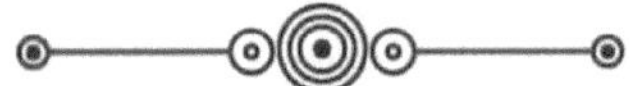

Once I was home from the hospital, the only thing on my to-do list was to rest and recuperate. After spending years in fight-or-flight mode, this sounded like an absolute dream. My mom made me a great big pot of chicken soup and a huge bowl of homemade mashed potatoes to eat over the next few days.

I also had developed quite an affinity for graham crackers, and my family kept me well-stocked in them. Again, being able to just eat without fearing the consequences was so amazing to me. Food could be comfort again. Eating those mashed potatoes felt like being wrapped in a warm blanket.

Almost as exciting as being able to eat without worry was the fact that I was finally able to get off of the cornucopia of medications that I had been taking for so long. I was able to successfully taper off of prednisone for the first time since the fall of 2007. My "moon face" quickly waned.

I was advised by Dr. Calvin, Dr. Stevens, and Mary to drink a ton of fluids to keep hydrated—all three of them stressed that a lot—and not just water, either. Gatorade and Powerade were encouraged as well. The colon is where a lot of your water and electrolytes are absorbed, and since I no longer had one, it would be very easy for me to become dehydrated. I had to overcompensate for this by drinking water and sports drinks as much as possible. I also found that products like Nuun and Liquid IV, which are powders that add extra electrolytes to water, were a great way to stay hydrated without the additional calories that come with sports drinks.

An ostomy nurse stopped by the house to assist me with changing the bag the first time, as well as to help me figure out what kind of supplies I wanted to use in the future. There was a much larger selection than I had ever imagined. I was also surprised to learn you didn't just go get ostomy bags at CVS or Walgreens. There was a mail-order company called Edgepark that would be my supplier from now on.

The ostomy nurse brought a catalog with her and showed me some different options. There were opaque ones, like the one I had first seen at Mary's office, and clear ones, like the one they sent me home wearing from the hospital. The nurse recommended starting out with the clear ones. It made it easier to see what you were doing when you put it on, as well as to see how much "output" you were getting. Once you got more accustomed to it, you could switch over to the opaque ones, she explained.

There were also one-piece and two-piece versions. This I already knew about from Brian from the support group, who had told me a lot about his own ostomy when I was first considering having surgery. With the one-piece version, the adhesive ring that affixes the bag to your skin is part of the ostomy bag itself. With the two-piece version, there was a separate "wafer" that adhered to your skin, and then you attached the bag to a flange on the wafer. The benefit of the two-piece system was that you could quickly change out the bag without having to redo the part that adhered to your skin.

Brian's recommendation was to go with the one-piece version. Fewer pieces meant fewer connections, he said, and less that could go wrong or leak. That made sense to me. I ended up going with the one-piece version based on his advice. I have never actually tried the two-piece version. I have heard some people say that an advantage of the two-piece version is if you play sports, you can get a smaller bag to give you a little more flexibility and range of motion while running around. Having the "wafer" stay on and only having to switch out the bag makes it easier to swap the bags out as needed. I agreed with Brian, that having only one piece felt like less opportunity for trouble.

The first couple of times I took a shower with the ostomy bag on felt weird. The nurse had assured me that it was okay to shower with it on and that it could get wet, but it made me anxious. I actually tried covering it by taping a small garbage bag over it, but that was even weirder; as the garbage bag got wet, it was weighed down and felt super heavy and awkward.

I ditched the garbage bag and then tried showering mostly facing away from the water so the ostomy bag didn't get wet, but that was weird too and made it hard to relax in the shower. I finally decided to just shower normally, and I got used to it pretty quickly. They were right, the bag could get wet and it didn't cause any issues.

Changing the ostomy bag in the shower became my preferred time to do it. I typically got anywhere from two to five days of wear time with a bag. I could tell it was due for a change because it would start to feel a little itchy around the stoma area. Gradually, the output wears away at the adhesive holding the bag to your skin. If you wait too long to change it, it starts to leak, and you really don't want that!

What I would usually do was get in the shower and have a garbage can right outside the tub. When I was almost done with the shower, I could remove the ostomy bag and throw it in the trash. Then I would have a chance to shower for a bit with no bag on, which felt really freeing. It also allowed me to wash the stoma and the area around it, which were usually covered by the bag.

I will say this: There were a few times early on that seeing and touching the stoma really freaked me out. I got in my own head thinking about the fact that this bright red thing sticking out of my abdomen was part of my intestine. *This is supposed to be inside me*, I would think. It would make me feel panicky. Ultimately, that feeling would subside. *Yeah*, I'd tell myself. *It used to be inside me… but the fact that it isn't anymore is what is letting me live a better life now. I would still be pooping in my pants if it wasn't for this.*

If you ever have an ostomy and you do take off your bag in the shower, make sure you dry the area thoroughly after you get out before you put on the new bag. I cannot stress that enough! I learned this the hard way early on. I was in such a hurry to get the new bag on that I put it on before I was dry. If you stick the new bag to wet skin, it won't adhere properly, and it will come loose. You'll end up with a bad leak before the day is done. Your skin needs to be nice and dry before you apply your next ostomy bag.

One thing I worried about was how to conceal the ostomy bag under my clothes. Would it be obvious that there was something there? I found a website called OstomySecrets that sold underwear specially designed for people with an ostomy. They sell boxer briefs, classic briefs, women's panties, and even wraps to wear when swimming that all cover and conceal the ostomy bag in a convenient, discreet pocket built into the waistline. This helps keep the bag from "bulging out," as it holds the bag much closer to your body.

This made me feel so much more comfortable and confident. My favorite time of year, though, is in the fall and winter, when I can layer up and throw on a nice loose sweater or hoodie, which makes it all but impossible to tell that there's a bag under my clothing. And even if people do notice it… I mean, really, who cares?

Oh, and for the record, the farting noises did stop. Most of the time the stoma is perfectly silent. There are some foods that can make it a little gassy, but they are the same foods that would do that to anyone. Broccoli, cabbage, dairy, carbonated drinks, stuff like that. As long as I avoid or eat those foods in moderation, my ileostomy is as quiet as the proverbial church mouse.

In the summer of 2010, Pam, Amanda, and I attended the annual Superman Celebration in Metropolis, Illinois. It was a three-day long festival in honor of the Man of Steel. There were special guests from Superman movies and TV shows, a trivia contest (I won a shirt!), people in costumes, and more. The town has a museum full of more memorabilia than you can imagine even exists. I was in heaven. The best part was, I didn't have to worry about the bathroom situation. The long car ride from New York to Illinois would have been damn near impossible in my prior condition, let alone just being able to walk around and enjoy the mostly outdoor festival itself. For the first time in years, I was able to actually do a fun activity without the constant worry of my symptoms spoiling everything. I felt "normal." And feeling normal was truly super.

I returned to work in June 2010 after an amazing and restorative period of rest and recuperation. There was still a spot waiting for me on my old team. The cubicle with my nameplate was still there, exactly as I had left it. I sat down and fired up my computer. For the first time in five years, I was ready to start a workday where I didn't have to worry about running to the bathroom. I could just focus on doing my job. I felt truly unstoppable.

Chapter Thirty-Five

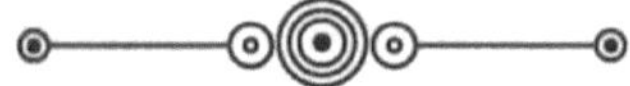

One day in October 2010, I felt some discomfort from behind the stoma. It felt kind of like something was stuck, even though output was still getting through. It just felt kind of irritated, like something behind or inside the stoma was getting sore. I called Dr. Calvin and told him what was going on.

"I'm going to have you go in and see Dr. Stevens," he said. "Let's have him take a look at your stoma and make sure there's not a blockage or any inflammation."

I called and made an appointment. Dr. Stevens was able to get me in for an office visit a couple of days later. He told me to bring an extra ostomy bag with me.

At the office visit, he said we could use the sigmoid scope again to look inside the stoma. He had me remove my current ostomy bag, which made me feel a bit nervous. He took the sigmoidoscopy scope and gently inserted it into the stoma. It was very surreal—I didn't feel a thing! There are no nerve endings there, so you don't feel any pain or anything. What a stark contrast to a few months earlier when he had barely been able to get the scope into my rectum because it was so inflamed and sensitive. It was very bizarre to be looking down at the exposed small intestine sticking out of my stomach and see the little scope going inside of it.

There was a monitor right next to us where Dr. Stevens and I could see what the camera on the end of the scope was picking up. After all of the colonoscopies that I had been sedated for—or woke up during but didn't have my glasses—this was my first time seeing my own guts in "real time." It was fascinating. It looked like an alien world.

"The good news is, I don't see any inflammation here," Dr. Stevens said. To be honest, even though it was only a couple of days later, I was already feeling better. Whatever had caused me that discomfort that prompted me to call Dr. Calvin seemed to have passed. "I'm going to take some biopsies while I'm in here," he continued. "It will take about a week to get the results back. But based on what I am seeing, I don't expect to find anything. It's possible that you just ate something that had you a little backed up, and that you had a small blockage that worked itself out on its own and just left things a little irritated."

"That's a relief," I said.

Dr. Stevens took some biopsies with the tiny little forceps on the end of the scope. This was the craziest thing I'd seen yet. I could see on the monitor that he was carefully cutting away some tissue, but I couldn't feel a thing. Then he slowly withdrew the scope.

"You did the right thing by coming in," Dr. Stevens said. "It's always better to be safe than sorry. You can go ahead and put your new ostomy bag on. I'll be in touch in a week or so about the results of the biopsies."

"Sounds good. Thank you so much, Dr. Stevens." I felt beyond grateful that I had found Dr. Calvin and Dr. Stevens. Between the two of them, I felt like I had an amazing medical support system now. I put on the new ostomy bag, which felt a little bit strange to do in his office since I usually did this after a shower. Then I headed home.

At the end of October, I got a letter in the mail from Dr. Stevens. I opened it.

Dear Mr. Dimino,

Your ileal biopsies from last week show very mild (microscopic only, as you may recall the visual appearance on the scope was quite normal) chronic active ileitis (inflammation). This is more consistent with Crohn's disease than ulcerative colitis and may require additional or ongoing treatment. You may wish to discuss this with Dr. Calvin; he has a copy of the biopsy result. If you have any questions, please do not hesitate to call.

I read the letter again. And again. And again. It didn't make sense, like I was reading something in a foreign language. It couldn't be saying what it seemed to be saying. They had told me that the final verdict was colitis. That was supposed to be case closed. I thought I was cured. They couldn't change it back to Crohn's now. They had to be wrong.

I leaned back against the wall. I slowly slid down it until I was sitting on the floor, still staring at the letter.

"I realize this is disappointing news," Dr. Calvin said at my office visit a few days later. "I know you're bummed. But let's look at the bright side. We are getting ahead of this after only a very, very mild flare-up. In fact, I would hesitate to even call it that. You had some slight inflammation that subsided on its own. What we want to do now is get you back on a maintenance drug to keep that from coming back. You tolerated 6-MP very well in the past. I want to have you do some bloodwork first so we can see how things are looking right now, and then I'd like to start you back on the 6-MP, which should keep you in remission."

Everything he was saying made sense. We were catching this early and after only a very minor incident. But the thought of getting back on any drug, even a mild one like 6-MP, seemed so unfair. I'd thought I was out of the woods. I had let myself believe that this was all over. I didn't want to get back on anything. Even going in for more bloodwork seemed like too much to ask. I'd had enough needles stuck in me for a lifetime.

But I didn't say any of that out loud.

"Okay," I said. "Sounds like a plan."

I walked out of Dr. Calvin's office and into the cool, crisp November afternoon. The few leaves that were still clinging to the trees were deep shades of red, orange, and yellow. Everything was cyclical after all. Something about the stillness of that afternoon was especially striking to me. I had just been given this awful news, and yet the world quietly went about its business. Was the universe's silent indifference to my troubles an insult being added to my injury, or a gentle reassurance of life's resilience? I wasn't sure yet.

I suppose it was fitting in a way. In the comics, the villain is never truly gone for good. The Joker always ends up escaping from the asylum. The Green Goblin miraculously rises from the dead. It was inevitable that my arch nemesis, the Crohn's demon, would come back to plague me again. I'd let myself believe that the nightmare was over, and finding out that it wasn't was a hard pill to swallow. But things were different now. I'd changed the game by getting the surgery. Now that I had the ostomy bag, the days of me running to the bathroom in a desperate attempt to avoid shitting my pants were over. The worst aspect of my disease had been literally cut out of me. The inflammation was coming back, but I could navigate that. Getting back on one medication was a lot better than having a regimen that covered my kitchen counter. I was discouraged, but I hadn't been defeated. I had gotten so much of my quality of life back since having the surgery. I hadn't let this disease beat me before, and I sure as hell wasn't going to let it beat me now.

I got the bloodwork done. I filled the 6-MP prescription.

And I prepared myself to keep fighting the never-ending battle.

Epilogue

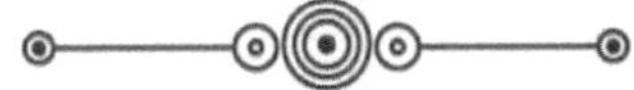

Idon't remember exactly when I stopped taking the 6-MP. I didn't discuss it with Dr. Calvin first. One day, I just stopped filling the prescription. I knew that with the diagnosis once again being Crohn's, there was a chance that the disease could come back. If it did, I figured we would cross that bridge when we got to it. Was that the most responsible thing to do? No, probably not. But I was tired of putting drugs into my body; I wanted to see what it would do if I left it to its own devices.

It's been more than ten years now, and I'm still in remission. I still haven't had a single flare-up since getting that letter from Dr. Stevens. That doesn't mean that I never will. Like my dad said, I just try to be thankful for every day that I feel good.

In the summer of 2012, Amanda and I welcomed our son, Dominic, into the world. I still remember the sound of his first cry so clearly. As the nurses weighed and measured our little bundle of joy, I talked soothingly to him.

"It's okay, little guy. It's okay. You're okay," I kept repeating. He kept wailing away anyway.

"It's normal for babies to cry like that when they are born," the nurse told me, thinking that my constant reassurances to him were a sign of concern. "It's actually a good thing."

"Oh, I know that," I said. "I just… I wish I could let him know that everything is going to be all right."

My mom had said in that email before my wedding that every parent wishes they could do better for their kids. I hadn't really understood that until this moment. Dominic had been in this world for only a few minutes so far, and I already wanted to comfort him and take away the fear and confusion he was feeling at being thrust into this strange new world.

In 2014, our second child, our daughter, Cora, made her entrance. Unlike her big brother, Cora cried only for a few moments, then settled down and seemed to already be looking at the world with wide-eyed wonder. Her calmness was such a stark contrast to her brother's birth. She looked up at me with an expression on her sweet little newborn face that seemed to say, "It's cool, Dad. I've got this." She seemed like an old soul, like she had somehow done this before. Wise beyond her years from minute one.

I have gotten so used to having the ostomy that it has become second nature. I do not regret having the surgery for a second. I think back to how intimidated I was by the ostomy when it was brand new, being kind of grossed out by it. Now I barely even think about it at all. But when I do, it actually comes with a feeling of gratitude. I am able to eat almost anything I want now, with a few specific exceptions: nuts, seeds, skins on things like potatoes or apples, lettuce, and popcorn are all too coarse and difficult to digest and can cause blockages, so I avoid those. (Yes, sadly, I still can't have popcorn at the movies, which sucks… but there are so many things that I can have now that I couldn't before that it doesn't bother me too much!) The quality of life that I have today is night and day compared to how it was when I was sick. The freedom that comes with not being tethered to the bathroom all the time is incredible. I've been able to go on vacations, socialize with friends, and just be present with my family without the stress of needing to constantly run to the restroom. I don't know how I would have been able to raise my kids while also battling my Crohn's symptoms. It's not an exaggeration to say that the surgery, in many ways, saved my life.

One of the challenges of writing this book was piecing together all of these events so long after the fact. I was very fortunate that I had access to many emails with my family, calendars, and day planners where I had kept track of all of my appointments, and lots of spiral notebooks where I would take notes during my doctor visits and write down what medications I was taking. This helped me so much in recreating the timeline of events. It would have been impossible without those records.

In one notebook, where I had written down details about insurance coverage, out-of-pocket maximums, deductibles, etcetera, I had plaintively scrawled in the margin: PLEASE MAKE ME BETTER! It was underlined several times, with a frown face drawn next to it. I didn't remember the moment that I wrote it, but I definitely remembered the feeling behind it.

Reading it so many years later, I felt like that note was calling out from somewhere in the past. From a time when I was still stuck, looking for answers, with no relief in sight. This Past Russ had documented so many things for me, so that I could write this book and share our story with others… but he was still suffering, still lost and feeling alone. I wished I could send something back to him, to help him. I wanted to comfort him, just like I had wanted to comfort my son in those first moments of his life.

I couldn't help myself. I picked up a pen, and right above the PLEASE MAKE ME BETTER! note, I wrote, I GOT YOU, BUDDY. WE'RE GOING TO BE OKAY.

I knew my note was not going to travel back in time to my past self so he could read it. But somehow I needed to add a sense of reassurance to that sad and lonely message.

To give a glimmer of hope where there once had been none.

Acknowledgements

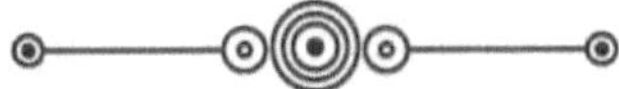

Thank you to Dr. Bill Valenti for being someone I could turn to when I was overwhelmed trying to navigate the medical world, as well as for your support of this book. I changed a lot of names in writing this thing, but I am proud to be able to include you in it by name.

Thank you to Dr. Calvin (that's not your real name, but you know who you are) for listening, caring, and getting me to where I am today. My quality of life is infinitely better now because of the tough decision that you helped me to make.

Thank you to the CCFA, the support group, and all the doctors, nurses, and researchers out there who dedicate their time, money, and effort to trying to make life more bearable for those who suffer from Crohn's and ulcerative colitis.

Thank you to my therapist, Theresa, for helping to get me through a pretty dark period of anxiety and depression that I experienced while working on this book, and for encouraging me to keep writing it because it was a story that needed to be told. Who knows, maybe I can cover my battle with depression in the sequel! (Just kidding… maybe.)

Thank you to April Randolph for showing me how to take those first steps toward actually publishing a book instead of just dreaming about it. You made me not only believe that I could do it, but understand how it could be done.

Thank you to Crystal Watanabe for her judicious edits. Much like my digestive tract, this book moved much more smoothly after cutting some things out of it!

Thank you to Carla Pinilla of Freaking Narnia for giving this book a final polish and making sure it was ready for a lot more eyes to see it.

Thank you to Richell Balansag for designing the cover of this book. You took my vague vision and brought it to life in an even better way than I had imagined.

Thank you to Abdul Rehman for creating the interior layout. You were instrumental in giving this book just the right look and feel, and I really appreciate your help.

Thank you to my parents for always supporting me. You taught me, Val, and Josh that we could do whatever we set our minds to. Now you have raised two published authors and an entrepreneur who took those lessons to heart. Thanks for always being our biggest fans. (And Mom, I'm sorry for all the swearing in this book.)

Thank you to my brother Josh. Our shared sense of humor has gotten me through a lot of tough times. Texting inside jokes back and forth always brightens my day. I take comfort in knowing that

I can text you "Who is your daddy and what does he do?" at any time of the day or night and you'll reply back "Sir, this is Hooters, you can't call here talking like that."

Thank you to my sister, Valerie, for your support, guidance, and encouragement in publishing this book. You blazed a trail for me to follow and I cannot thank you enough for that. Even though you are my little sister, sometimes I'm the one who looks up to you. And for anyone out there who thinks that I'm a good writer, you really should check out Val's book, *The Man Behind the Curtain* – she is a way more gooder writer than me!

Thank you to Amanda for standing by me through all of it. Let's admit it, when we said, "in sickness and in health," you really drew the short end of the stick…! But you never made me feel like a burden. This book is the story of a journey that we took together, and I could not have done it on my own. I am so grateful for your unwavering support. I love you so much.

Thank you to Dominic and Cora, for being the best kids I could have ever asked for, as well as for putting up with my corny jokes. You both have so much creativity, intelligence, humor, and thoughtfulness to offer the world. Take that spark inside of you and do whatever you want with it. Your mom and I will be cheering you on. Always.

Last but not least, thank you to you. The person reading this book. I am guessing that you or someone that you care about has Crohn's, ulcerative colitis, or some other form of IBS or IBD. I hope sharing my story made you realize that you're not alone. I hope you find relief soon, and that in the meantime you find a way to hold on to the good moments. I'm rooting for you.

About The Author

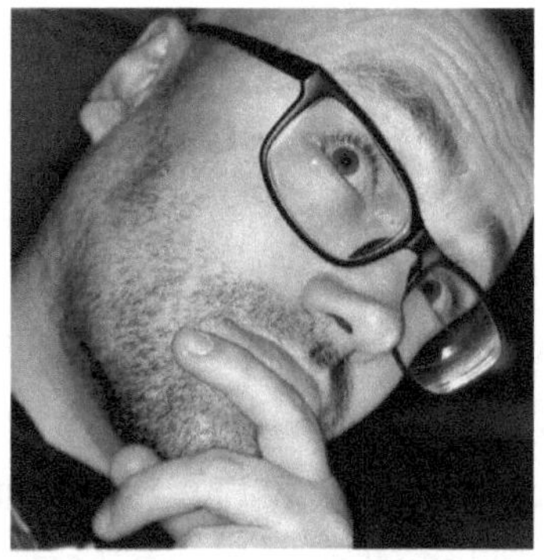

Russ Dimino wants you to know that he was a nerd before it was cool to be one. He learned to read at an early age thanks in large part to *Incredible Hulk* comic books. He has written many columns for KryptonSite, a renowned website dedicated to Superman-related television shows. He lives in Rochester, New York, with his wife Amanda and their children Dominic and Cora. This is his first book.

https://www.russdimino.com

Author Photo by Cora Dimino

www.ingramcontent.com/pod-product-compliance
Lightning Source LLC
Chambersburg PA
CBHW031115160726
47991CB00004B/1389